Data Interpretation for Paediatric

Data Interpretation for Paediatric Examinations

Christopher O'Callaghan
B Med Sci BM BS MRCP
Senior Lecturer in Child Health, University of Leicester; Honorary Consultant, Leicester Royal Infirmary, Leicester, UK

Terence Stephenson
BSc BM MCh MRCP
Senior Lecturer in Child Health, University of Nottingham; Honorary Consultant; Queen's Medical Centre, Nottingham, UK

CHURCHILL LIVINGSTONE
EDINBURGH LONDON MADRID MELBOURNE NEW YORK AND TOKYO 1994

CHURCHILL LIVINGSTONE
Medical Division of Longman Group UK Limited

Distributed in the United States of America by Churchill
Livingstone Inc., 650 Avenue of the Americas, New York,
N.Y. 10011, and by associated companies, branches and
representatives throughout the world.

First published 1994

ISBN 0-443-05010-4

British Library Cataloguing in Publication Data
A catalogue record for this book is available from the
British Library.

Library of Congress Cataloging in Publication Data
A catalog record for this book is available from the
Library of Congress.

The
publisher's
policy is to use
**paper manufactured
from sustainable forests**

Produced by Longman Singapore Publishers (Pte) Ltd.
Printed in Singapore.

Acknowledgement

Kath Walters typed much of the manuscript. Margaret Barrow, Hugh Kelso, David Mellor, Connie Pullan and Nick Rutter provided initial drafts for some of the questions. We are extremely grateful to Peter Barry and Derek Johnston who offered valuable comments on the manuscript. Any remaining errors are our fault entirely. We would be delighted to hear from anyone wishing to point out mistakes or alternative answers which we have overlooked.

Contents

Introduction

In 1972, the three Royal Colleges of Physicians of the United Kingdom introduced a common Part II examination for the Membership of the Royal College of Physicians, MRCP(UK). Since 1977, candidates have been able to sit the Part II examination in either general medicine or paediatrics.

To qualify for the second part of the MRCP examination in paediatrics, the candidate must fulfil three criteria. First, he/she must have passed the Part I (multiple choice examination) of the MRCP(UK), unless holding one of the diplomas giving exemption from Part I (see *Examination Regulations and Information for Candidates*, available from any of the Royal Colleges). From October 1993, there has been the option of taking the Part I multiple choice paper in paediatrics. Fifty per cent of questions are common to the general medicine Part I option and both options devote roughly half the paper to basic science and half to clinical disorders. Areas of basic science which are particularly important for the paediatric Part I are genetics, embryology, fetal and child physiology, growth and development, and child and family psychology. The candidate has a maximum of four attempts and must pass the second part within 7 years of obtaining the Part I. There is full reciprocity between the paediatric and general Part I in allowing successful candidates to proceed to either option at Part II, and this is unlikely to change. However, this reciprocity also holds for the number of failures allowed at Part I (i.e. only four attempts in all).

The second criterion is that the candidate must have been fully registered for at least 18 months (i.e. usually 2.5 years from graduation) and spent not < 12 months caring for adult or paediatric emergencies after registration. Finally, the candidate must be sponsored by two Fellows of a Royal College of Physicians (Royal College of Australasia is acceptable) or members of a Royal Colleges of Physicians of > 8 years' standing. There are three Royal Colleges of Physicians in the United Kingdom (London, Edinburgh and Glasgow). The candidate need not sit Parts I and II with the same College. If a candidate fails either the written or clinical sections of Part II, he/she must re-take the whole examination. A maximum of six attempts are allowed (three at one College, two at another, one at the last) and the written and clinical sections of the Part II examination must be taken with the same College. Exactly the same paper is used at a given sitting, whether in London, Edinburgh, Glasgow or elsewhere in the world. There is no evidence that the clinical examination is easier in one or other of the Colleges. The pass rate remains remarkably consistent but varies by a small amount between each College on every sitting and no one College has a consistently higher or lower pass rate.

The Part II examination for MRCP (UK) consists of written, oral and clinical sections and the written examination precedes the oral and clinical examinations by about 6 weeks. The candidate must pass, or achieve a borderline pass, in the written examination before he/she is invited to attend for the clinical and oral examinations.

The written section of the Part II examination consists of three papers (see Table 1), all of which are taken on the same day at one of the Royal Colleges and also in Hong Kong, Oman, Malaysia, Saudi Arabia and Kuwait. These papers are based on case histories (also known as grey cases), photographs or 'printed material' (which were previously projected as slides but are now given in a small booklet) and data interpretation questions. The case history examination consists of four or more compulsory questions for which 55 minutes are allowed. One question is common to both the adult and paediatric papers. The grey cases normally include one extended case history which is composed of up to nine sections and may involve 'multi-media' presentation (e.g. growth charts, X-rays, pathological slides, electrocardiographs, data). There are 20 items of printed material which may include clinical photographs, blood films and retinal photographs and 40 minutes are allowed for this paper. This book deals only with answering data interpretation questions. The data interpretation examination paper contains 10 compulsory questions based on laboratory or graphical data and Table 2 lists questions which have appeared in recent years. Two of the questions are common to the adult and paediatric examinations. Forty-five minutes are allowed for this paper. All three parts of the written examination are compulsory and the candidate has no choice over

Table 1 Format of the Paediatric MRCP(UK) Part II Examination

Category	Content	Time (min)	% final mark
Case histories ('Grey cases')	Tests ability to analyse clinical data, exclude unimportant findings, recognize emergencies, consider differential diagnoses, decide further investigations and form a management plan. Four or five cases with an *average* total mark per case of 8. Individual questions can score more or fewer than 8. For example, the extended case history scores more marks	55	33.3
Photographic material	Clinical, radiological or haematological slides with a brief stem of one or two sentences to give the clinical background. A pair of photographs may be used to illustrate a single question (e.g. an X-ray with a clinical photograph of the same patient). 20 questions with an *average* total mark per photograph of 4	40	33.3
Data interpretation	Tests ability to assess the result of investigations in a clinical setting. Ten questions with an *average* total mark per question of 5	45	33.3

Table 2 Previous data interpretation topics used in the MRCP (UK) examination

1. Pedigree of vitamin D-resistant rickets and probability of child being affected
2. Cerebrospinal fluid and electrolytes — tuberculous meningitis and inappropriate secretion of antidiuretic hormone
3. Audiogram
4. Urea and electrolytes = Addison's disease
5. Urea and electrolytes and a water deprivation test = psychogenic polydipsia
6. Coagulation results
7. Neonatal blood gas
8. Developmental milestones
9. Blood gas = salicylate ingestion
10. Full blood count = β-thalassaemia trait

1. Full blood count = aplastic anaemia
2. Cerebrospinal fluid and urea and electrolytes = bacterial meningitis and inappropriate secretion of antidiuretic hormone
3. Electrocardiogram = Wolff-Parkinson-White syndrome
4. Cerebrospinal fluid = cerebral abscess
5. Blood gas = respiratory acidosis and compensatory metabolic alkalosis (as a result of Pierre Robin syndrome)
6. Urea and electrolytes, blood gas and cerebrospinal fluid from a neonate with seizures
7. Urea and electrolytes = uric acid nephropathy and renal failure due to tumour lysis syndrome
8. Full blood count = twin–twin transfusion
9. Pedigree, what are probabilities of offspring being affected?
10. Electrocardiogram = ventricular tachycardia

1. Liver function tests = Reye's syndrome
2. Blood gas = salicylate overdose
3. Clotting studies = heparin-contaminated sample
4. Growth chart = neglect
5. Electrocardiogram = pulmonary hypertension due to obstructed upper airway
6. Blood and urine protein = congenital nephrotic
7. Blood results = hypoparathyroidism
8. Blood gas and history = inborn error of metabolism
9. Urea and electrolytes = tumour lysis syndrome
10. Lung function tests = asthma

1. Electroencephalogram = petit mal epilepsy
2. Electrocardiogram = ostium primum atrial septal defect
3. Tympanogram = bilateral sensory neural deafness
4. Blood gas = compensated respiratory acidosis
5. Electrolytes = diabetes insipidus
6. Full blood count = Fanconi's anaemia
7. Electrolytes = renal tubular acidosis
8. Full blood count = infectious mononucleosis
9. Nitrogen wash-out test = congenital heart disease

1. Cerebrospinal fluid = tuberculous meningitis
2. Blood results = ABO-incompatible neonatal jaundice
3. Electrolytes = pyloric stenosis
4. Electroencephalogram = hypsarrhythmia
5. Developmental milestones
6. Audiogram
7. Blood gas = mixed respiratory metabolic acidosis
8. Urine and blood electrolytes = renal glycosuria
9. Full blood count = Von Willebrand's disease

which questions he/she may answer. The candidate must attempt to answer all questions.

It is apparent from Table 2 that the examiners may ask about a wide range of data and, in addition to requesting the underlying diagnosis, may also ask for further investigations or treatment in a subsidiary question. If the answer to the first part of the question is wrong, then often no marks can be obtained even if the answer to the subsidiary question is correct. For example, consider a question requiring two answers, (a) the diagnosis and (b) an appropriate investigation. If a candidate's answer to the first part of the question is wrong and scores 0, then a correct investigation for this suggested diagnosis is also wrong and scores 0. If the answer to (a) is not totally wrong and scores 1 out of 4 marks, then an appropriate answer to (b) will be scaled down similarly. Occasionally, an incorrect answer to (a), marked 0, requires the same investigation in (b) as for a correct diagnosis. In these circumstances, the full mark for (b) will be given.

It is very rare for an identical question to appear but there are recurring themes. For example, candidates are expected to be very familiar with interpretation of urea and electrolytes, full blood counts, arterial blood gases, cerebrospinal fluid, coagulation results and electrocardiograms. This does not seem unreasonable as these are investigations which are in common use in both outpatient paediatrics and in relation to children admitted acutely; a registrar holding the MRCP(UK) qualification would be expected to have a sound working knowledge of this type of data. Questions involving electrocardiograms or cardiac catheterization data, karyotypes or family pedigrees, developmental milestones, electroencephalograms, audiograms and growth charts also occur fairly frequently. It is possible that data incorporating a visual component (e.g. a corresponding clinical photograph) may be introduced into the examination in the future but no significant changes are planned, at least as far as 1995.

Marking of the written section

Examiners from each College are responsible for the marking of one of the question papers of each candidate, irrespective of a candidate's College of entry. Every question is marked independently from the others. Each answer is marked again by another examiner, to make sure that no errors have been made by the original marker. Candidates are entirely anonymous as far as the examiners are concerned. The examiner will not know how many previous attempts the candidate has had at the examination, whether he/she has failed the written examination before or how he/she has done in another part of the examination. Although the total raw marks for each paper are different (see Table 1), all three papers are given equal weight in the final analysis. The final mark for each candidate is then the sum of all three papers. In order to pass, therefore, it is not necessary to obtain a pass mark in all three parts of the written examination, provided the total mark reaches the required pass mark. Each candidate is given a total mark for the written examination out of 20.

About 75% of candidates who sit the written examination on any one day will be allowed to progress to the clinical examinations. Of this 75%, 60% will have obtained a mark of >10 out of 20 and therefore have a clear pass in the written examination. The other 15% will have been marked with a 9 out of 20, which is a borderline pass in the written examination. A candidate who gains 9 in the written section will be required to gain 3 extra marks in either the oral or clinical examinations to pass. In essence, a candidate with a bare fail in the written examination must obtain a total of 27 out of 50 in the whole of the Part II examination to pass, as opposed to a candidate who passes the written examination who must obtain a straightforward 25 out of 50 to pass overall. Approximately 15% of candidates with a borderline 9 from the written examination will pass the clinical exam with sufficient marks to obtain the MRCP(UK). The relationship between the marking in the written examination and the various parts of the clinical examination is described in more detail in *Clinical Paediatrics for Postgraduate Examinations*, 2nd edn. (Stephenson & Wallace 1995).

The remaining 25% of the original cohort who obtain a mark of 8 or below in the written section are eliminated from the rest of the examination. All the candidates who fail the written examination receive notification of their mark out of 20 and whether they have passed or failed each of the three sections of the written exam. Counselling is not offered after a fail in the written exam. A candidate who scores a very poor mark in the clinical and oral examination may be strongly recommended not to re-enter the exam for 6–12 months. They may also be referred to a senior Fellow of one of the Colleges for counselling.

Tactics on answering data interpretation questions

The examination has been designed to require minimal writing to allow for objective marking by the examiners. The markers try to decipher candidate's handwriting but if writing is not legible, then no marks can be obtained. (If you are in doubt about whether your writing is legible, always print your answer in block capitals.) Some candidates have suggested that poor handwriting was the reason for failure in the written examination but this has never been the sole reason for failure.

Marks are awarded by the examiners in a pre-determined manner and quite specific answers are required. It is therefore vital that candidates listen carefully to the instructions given by the invigilator and re-read the questions carefully before they answer. Since specific answers are required, it is of no avail to attempt to explain your thoughts to the examiners. The answer will be either right or wrong, and if wrong no amount of special pleading will persuade the examiner to change his mind! Answers should be precise, as vague answers can score significantly lower marks. For example, in answering questions about clinical photographs, always specify whether it is the child's right or left side which is abnormal. A data interpretation question which asks for a karyotype should not be answered with 'Turner's syndrome'. The correct answer would be 45 XO. If the correct answer to a question is allergic bronchopulmonary aspergillosis and the candidate writes only bronchopulmonary aspergillosis, the omission of the word allergic may cost as much as half the marks.

Each question will ask for a specific number of answers, such as the two most likely diagnoses or the two most useful investigations. Correct answers to this question will receive maximum marks but since there is sometimes more than one possible correct answer, marks are awarded on a scale according to their correspondence with a panel of answers previously decided by the examining board. For example, the two best answers would receive maximum marks but lower marks would be awarded for other reasonable diagnoses. However, where the best answer is obviously much better than the others, the difference in marks between the best and the other answers would be correspondingly greater. The weighting of the preferential answers varies from one question to another and therefore all the data interpretation questions are not necessarily of equal value. No credit will be given for answers which exceed the number required. Such additional answers will be ignored. If the two most likely diagnoses were requested and the candidate's third answer is the best, he/she will obtain no marks for that and indeed may obtain fewer marks for the previous two answers given.

Examples

Suppose that the data clearly show that a child is suffering from nephrogenic diabetes insipidus. In answer to the question 'What is the most likely cause of these biochemical findings?', the marker's answer key might be as follows:

4 marks   Nephrogenic diabetes insipidus

3 marks   Diabetes insipidus

2 marks   Renal tubular defect

1 mark   Overconcentrated feed

0 marks   Renal failure

Total maximum = 4 marks

A subsequent question about cerebrospinal fluid findings in a child with weakness may be 'What is the clinical diagnosis?'; the answer key might be as follows:

2 marks   Acute poliomyelitis

1 mark   Poliomyelitis

0 marks   Guillain-Barré syndrome

'Which further investigation may help confirm the diagnosis?'

2 marks   Throat swab for viral culture

2 marks   Stool for viral culture

2 marks   Blood sample for acute viral titres

1 mark   Throat swab

0 marks   Blood culture

'What abnormality would be found on spirometry?'

2 marks   Restrictive lung defect

2 marks   Reduced forced vital capacity

0 marks   Obstructive lung defect

Total maximum = 6 marks

The examiners recognize the difficulty posed by multiple tests (e.g. full blood count; urea and electrolytes; urine or cerebrospinal fluid microscopy, culture and sensitivity) and this causes much confusion to candidates. The yardstick which the examiners apply is whether these tests are usually requested simultaneously in normal practice. There is little variation between hospitals in this and the three examples given above are usually requested together routinely in all hospitals in the UK. In contrast, for example, full blood count and erythrocyte sedimentation rate would be separate investigations in most hospitals, as would urea and electrolytes and liver functions tests, or electrocardiogram and echocardiograph.

All data are presented using SI units, including blood gases which are given in kPa (1 kPa is approximately equal to 7.5 mmHg). The candidate is expected to know the normal ranges for common laboratory values (e.g. urea and electrolytes, red blood cell indices, white cell counts, platelet counts and intervals on the electrocardiogram). The normal ranges for less common investigations, such as endocrine assays which are often done by supra-regional laboratories, will be given.

There is *no* negative marking in any part of the written section of the Part II MRCP(UK) examination. The candidate should therefore answer *all* questions. If you are not sure, there is nothing to be lost by guessing. Occasionally, 'normal', 'no treatment' or 'reassure' are all acceptable answers. When asked for further investigations or treatment, always try to think of those things you would do first in the clinical setting and which are simplest and least expensive, rather than opting for esoteric investigations. Finally, remember that if your answer to the first part of the question is wrong, the second part may score no marks even if correct, so do read the question very carefully and try to get the first part right at least.

Using this book

The questions presented in this book reflect the style and broadly the standard of the real examination. The questions have been grouped as in the examination papers, 10 questions at a time, and within each group there are one or two more difficult questions to push the candidate to the limit. The answers are given at the end of each paper and we would advise that the candidate attempts each set of 10 questions as a paper before looking at any of the answers. It is very easy to convince yourself that you are doing well by flicking back and forth between the questions and answers. In some questions, the answers are ranked according to their acceptability, e.g.

Acquired aplastic anaemia   — best answer

Bone marrow failure   ⎫   — correct but less
Fanconi's anaemia   ⎬   appropriate than
Schwachman–Diamond syndrome   ⎭   above

Pancytopenia   — least acceptable answer

(see p. 21)

We have included some 'trick' questions which require some lateral thinking. Although the examining boards try to avoid setting misleading or ambiguous questions, similar questions have appeared in the examination and are not really 'trick' questions in the sense that the data interpretation is supposed to mimic real practice and in this situation the numbers are not always what they seem. Some questions have been included which are unlikely to appear in the real examination but which we judge make valuable teaching points about the interpretation of data generally. Sometimes the understanding of difficult metabolic and endocrine disorders can be advanced more by the answering of questions than by reading weighty tomes on the subject!

Many of the questions in this book have been honed by using them on revision courses for candidates preparing for the MRCP(UK). We have also canvassed the views of these candidates on how a revision book on data interpretation could be best written and we hope this book will help you. We have done our utmost to ensure that the information in this introductory chapter is factually correct as it is important that candidates are not mislead by 'Membership mythology'. Good luck!

References

Chin KC, Tarlow MJ 1989 Paediatric revision. Churchill Livingstone, Edinburgh
Examination Regulations and Information for Candidates for the MRCP(UK), 1993. Available from:

Royal College of Physicians of Edinburgh,
9, Queen Street,
Edinburgh EH2 1JQ
Tel: 031–225 7324

Royal College of Physicians and Surgeons of Glasgow,
224 St. Vincent Street,
Glasgow G2 5RJ
Tel: 041–221 6072

Royal College of Physicians of London,
11 St. Andrew's Place,
Regent's Park,
London NW1 4LE
Tel: 071–935 1174

Stephenson T, Wallace H 1995 Clinical paediatrics for postgraduate
examinations, 2nd edn. Churchill Livingstone, Edinburgh

Paper 1 QUESTIONS

Question 1.1

This is the audiogram from an 8-year-old boy. His mother was worried by his hearing. He had passed his routine audiometry screen at 5 years and there was no family history of ear problems. On examination no abnormalities were found.

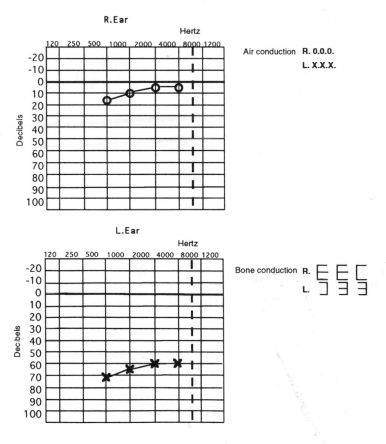

1. What type of hearing loss is this likely to be?
2. What is the most likely cause?

Question 1.2

Overleaf is the ECG from a 7-year-old African boy.

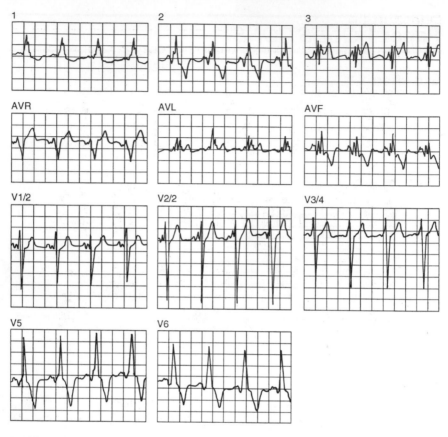

1. What does the ECG show?
2. Comment on the evidence of ventricular hypertrophy in this ECG.

Question 1.3

These are the cardiac catheter results of a newborn child.

	Oxygen saturation (%)	Blood pressure (mmHg) (systolic/diastolic)
Right atrium	35	
Right ventricle	35	80/7
Pulmonary artery	95	58/8
Left atrium	95	
Left ventricle	95'	58/8
Aorta	35	85/60

1. What is the diagnosis?

Question 1.4

Chromosomal analysis revealed the following karyotype in a 3-month-old girl.

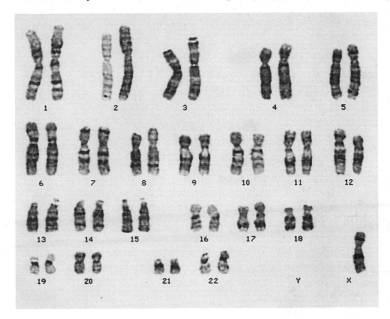

1. What is the diagnosis?
2. In the long term, is the child likely to have an IQ above 80?
3. Untreated, is the girl's final height likely to be within the normal range for adult women?
4. Give two drugs this child will probably receive?

Question 1.5

A woman gives birth to a 3.8 kg infant at 36 weeks gestation after leaking clear liquor for 3 days. The baby is well until 24 h later when he starts to grunt and is found to be centrally cyanosed. Arterial blood gases in air results are:

pH   7.19
PaO_2 6.9 kPa
$PaCO_2$ 5.2 kPa

The infant is intubated and commenced on positive pressure ventilation. A chest X-ray shows bilateral generalized opacification. The tip of the nasogastic tube is in the stomach. The heart size is normal on chest X-ray and an echocardiogram shows normal cardiac anatomy and vascular connections.

1. What is the most likely diagnosis?
2. What single investigation will be most helpful in confirming this?

Question 1.6

A 6½-year-old child started school at 5 years and has recently had recurrent upper respiratory tract infections and lethargy. Prior to this, he was perfectly well. Full blood count gives the following results:

Haemoglobin	8.0 g/dl
Platelet count	$80 \times 10^9/l$
White cell count	$4.0 \times 10^9/l$
Red cell count	$3.8 \times 10^{12}/l$
Reticulocytes	0.5% of total red cell count
Bone marrow biopsy	No malignant cells

1. What is the most likely diagnosis?

Question 1.7

A registrar took several minutes to obtain a blood sample from a well 18-month-old child in casualty. The following laboratory results were obtained:

Haemoglobin	16 g/dl
Calcium	2.9 mmol/l
Total protein	80 g/l
Albumin	45 g/l
Blood glucose	4.0 mmol/l

Blood was re-taken by a senior house officer 1 h later and the following results were obtained:

Haemoglobin	14.1 g/dl
Calcium	2.3 mmol/l
Total protein	70 g/l
Albumin	38 g/l
Blood glucose	4.0 mmol/l

Both samples were taken with the child lying supine.

1. What is the most likely explanation for the change in results when blood was taken 1 h later?

Question 1.8

A 13-year-old boy investigated for general malaise was noted to have hilar lymphadenopathy on chest X-ray examination. The following laboratory results were obtained:

Calcium	3.0 mmol/l
AS transferase	15 U/l
Protein	77 g/l
Albumin	45 g/l
Angiotensin converting enzyme	114 nmol/l/min (normal 14–41 nmol/l/min)

1. What is the most likely diagnosis?
2. Give two further investigations that may help confirm your diagnosis.

Question 1.9

A 4-year-old boy was referred to an orthopaedic clinic because of 'knock knees'. The following blood results were obtained:

Alkaline phosphatase	Increased
Serum phosphate	Decreased
Calcium	Low/normal range
CRP	2 mg/l
Plasma 25 hydroxycholecalciferol	Decreased
Serum parathyroid hormone	Increased/normal

1. What is the most likely diagnosis?
2. Give four other clinical features that may be seen.

Question 1.10

A well looking child was investigated for intermittent hypoglycaemia. This was not related to periods of fasting. The following results were obtained during a typical attack:

Blood glucose	1.2 mmol/l
Insulin	Elevated
Ketones	Absent in serum and urine
C-peptide	Suppressed

1. What is the likely cause of the child's hypoglycaemia?

Paper 1 *ANSWERS*

Answer 1.1

1. Profound (or severe) sensorineural deafness affecting the left ear

   Sensorineural deafness affecting the left ear

   Profound sensorineural deafness

   Sensorineural deafness

2. Mumps infection after 5 years of age

   Sensorineural deafness due to viral infection
   Progressive hereditary deafness
   Acoustic neuroma

Discussion

The audiogram gives data for air conduction only. The degree of hearing loss (>60 dcb) and the fact that it affects all frequencies demonstrates that it is too severe to be a conductive hearing loss. It is also obvious from the audiogram that it is unilateral and as the history gives no mention of abnormality of the external ear or drum, the condition has been acquired.

In general terms, a loss of >50 dcb is extremely unlikely to be due to conductive deafness and this ear is probably completely deaf; the response at 70 dcb is a 'shadow' via bone conduction to the good right ear. This represents profound acquired left sensorineural deafness and the most likely cause is mumps.

Answer 1.2

1. Left bundle branch block
2. A diagnosis of ventricular hypertropy should not be made when left bundle branch block is present. QRS voltages may be greater than normal because of the asynchrony of depolarization of each ventricle

Discussion

On brief inspection of an ECG of a child with left bundle branch block, the QRS looks like an 'M' in 1 or V6 and a 'W' in AVR or V1. The generally accepted criteria for left bundle branch block include:

— a QRS duration longer than the upper limits of normal for the patient's age;
— left axis deviation for the patient's age;
— loss of Q waves in leads 1, V5 and V6;
— slurred and wide R waves in 1, AVL, V5 and V6;

— wide S waves in V1 and V2;
— ST depression and T wave inversion in V4, V5 and V6 is common;
— QRS voltages may be greater than normal.

Further reading

*Park M K, Guntheroff W G 1992 How to read pediatric ECGs, 2nd edn.
Mosby Yearbook, St Louis*

Answer 1.3

1. Transpostion of the great arteries

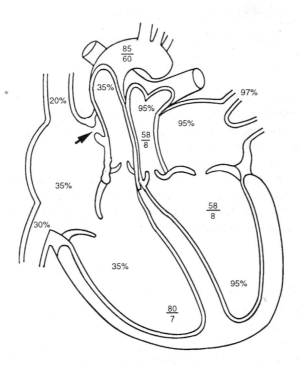

Discussion

Complete transposition of the great arteries is a common cardiac abnormality found in approximately 5% of all children with congenital heart disease. The aorta originates from the morphological right ventricle and the pulmonary artery from the morphological left ventricle. The consequence of this is that unoxygenated systemic venous blood, returning to the heart, passes through the right atrium and right ventricle and is ejected into the aorta. Similarly, oxygenated pulmonary venous blood reaches the left side of the heart and is returned to the pulmonary artery. The clinical presentation is characterized by severe and life-threatening hypoxaemia early in life. The presence or absence of associated cardiac abnormalities dictates presentation, clinical course and surgical treatment.

To allow life, there must be some means of mixing of blood between the two circulations. In neonates with transposition of the great arteries and an intact ventricular septum, a foramen ovale or atrial septal defect is usually present, helping exchange of blood at the atrial level. Presence of a patent ductus arteriosus will enhance this exchange. Unfortunately, the patent ductus arteriosus closes physiologically within a few days of birth. The closure of the duct may precipitate a dramatic change in the clinical appearance of the newborn, from being apparently healthy to showing intense cyanosis.

Patients with transposition of the great arteries and a significant ventricular septal defect have a different clinical picture. They often have adequate exchange of blood with mixing at both atrial and ventricular levels. Only mild cyanosis may be present in the early neonatal period, and a cardiovascular anomaly is often not suspected until a few weeks later. These patients may present with congestive heart failure towards the end of the first month of life because of the large ventricular septal defect.

The third main category of patients is those with a complex transposition. This involves complete transposition, ventricular septal defect and a varying degree of left ventricular outflow tract obstruction. The balance between pulmonary and systemic blood flows is dependent upon the degree of pulmonary stenosis. When this is severe, or if pulmonary atresia exists, patients present with cyanosis and reduced pulmonary blood flow early in life. However, if the degree of pulmonary stenosis is less severe, clinical presentation may be due to the presence of cyanosis and/or the detection of a heart murmur. This presentation may occur late in infancy. With cross-sectional echocardiography, it is possible to demonstrate the atrioventricular and ventriculoatrial connections reliably, thus enabling the diagnosis of transposition of the great arteries. Though catheterization will confirm the diagnosis and reveal the presence and significance of associated abnormalities, the major indication for catheterization is to perform balloon atrial septostomy.

Further reading
Campbell A G M, McIntosh N (eds) 1992 Forfar and Arneil's Textbook of paediatrics, 4th edn. Churchill Livingstone, Edinburgh, pp. 658–690

Answer 1.4

1. Turner's syndrome (45 XO karyotype)
2. Yes
3. No
4. Growth hormone
   Phased introduction of oestrogens

Discussion

Loss of a sex chromosome (i.e. 45 XO) is a common finding in abortus material and only around 3–5% of conceptions survive to third trimester. The incidence in liveborn female infants is 1 in 5000.

Turner's syndrome may be detected during antenatal ultrasonography by generalized hydrops or swelling of the subcutaneous tissue over the neck. The excess of tissue fluid is due to delayed maturation of the lymphatic drainage system. In surviving babies, the vestiges of this intrauterine oedema manifest as residual neck webbing, puffy hands and feet and small hyperconvex nails. Fifteen per cent of cases have coarctation of the aorta.

Short stature is the most common presenting feature in childhood. Patients are born short, and a progressive fall in growth velocity during the early years means the final height of untreated patients is about 142 cm (SD 6 cm). (The third centile for the normal adult female population in the UK is about 150 cm.) Short stature is treated with growth hormone.

Examination may also reveal a low posterior hairline, increased carrying angles of the arms, widely spaced nipples (shield chest) and Madelung deformity of the wrists.

Intelligence is frequently normal in patients with Turner's syndrome, the distribution curve of IQ being shifted a little lower than in the general population. However, the overlap is such that an academic career is not precluded, in contrast to some of the other sex chromosome abnormalities.

Presentation in adult life is with primary amenorrhoea and infertility. In Turner's syndrome the ovaries develop normally during the first half of intrauterine life. Thereafter, they regress (ovarian dysgenesis), leaving only small strands of ovarian tissue (streak gonads). Treatment with genetically engineered oestrogen replacement therapy should be commenced at around the time of onset of puberty.

Further reading

Hull D, Johnston D I 1993 Essential paediatrics, 3rd edn. Churchill Livingstone, Edinburgh, p. 18

Answer 1.5

1. Group B streptococcal pneumonia

   Congenital pneumonia

   ('Sepsis' or 'infection' are too vague)

2. Blood culture

   Urine for streptococcal antigen
   Lumbar puncture

Discussion

The infant has parenchymal lung disease resulting in Type 1 respiratory failure (hypoxia but normocapnia) associated with a metabolic acidosis. The maturity of the infant, the 'stress' of prolonged (i.e. >24 h) rupture of the membranes and the delay in onset of symptoms do not support hyaline membrane disease as the cause of the respiratory distress, despite the radiological appearances. Because of the difficulty in differentiating Group B streptococcal pneumonia from hyaline membrane disease on chest X-ray, all infants with respiratory distress which is not due to a congenital abnormality should be started on intravenous benzyl penicillin. The chest X-ray effectively excludes diaphragmatic hernia, oesophageal atresia and congenital heart disease, all of which may present after an initial 'honeymoon period'. The prolonged rupture of the membranes increases the risk of congenital pneumonia acquired by ascending infection from the genital tract. Maternal fever, vaginal discharge, offensive liquor (suggesting listeria) or active cervicitis (suggesting herpes) would increase suspicion of a congenital infection.

The nomenclature of streptococci often leads to confusion. Streptococci are divided into three groups depending on the degree of haemolysis caused when cultured on blood agar (e.g. *Streptococcus faecalis* produces no haemolytic effect; *Streptococcus viridans* causes partial or α-haemolysis; *Streptococcus pyogenes* causes complete or β-haemolysis). β-haemolytic streptococci can be further classified. Group A streptococci are the commonest cause of human streptococcal infection (e.g. tonsillitis). Group B streptococci are pathogenic in the newborn and a virulent cause of neonatal pneumonia, septicaemia and meningitis. Both early onset (within days of birth) and late onset (>1 week after birth) neonatal illnesses are recognized. There is a high mortality even with prompt recognition and appropriate treatment.

A full blood count may show neutropenia or leucocytosis in Group B streptococcal infection but will not alter management or provide a definitive microbiological diagnosis. Group B streptococcus is a common commensal in the vagina of many pregnant women and therefore the culture of the organism from surface swabs taken from the baby does not confirm pathogenicity. Similarly, the infant's gastric aspirate will not be sterile after 24 h, even in a healthy neonate, so the presence of Gram-positive cocci on microscopy (or the rapid confirmation of streptococcal antigen by counterimmune electrophoresis) is not diagnostic either. Couterimmune electrophoresis may detect streptococcal antigen in the urine but collection of urine in the newborn is not always reliable and should not delay the start of antibiotics. Blood cultures obtained before antibiotics are commenced give a high positive detection rate in Group B streptococcal infection: if another pathogen is cultured, then antibiotic therapy can be modified accordingly (e.g. ampicillin and gentamicin are synergistic against *Listeria monocytogenes*).

Further reading

Campbell A G M, McIntosh N (eds) 1992 *Forfar and Arneil's Textbook of paediatrics*, 4th edn. Churchill Livingstone, Edinburgh, pp. 1385–1388

Answer 1.6

1. Acquired aplastic anaemia

Bone marrow failure
Fanconi's anaemia
Schwachman–Diamond syndrome

Pancytopenia

Discussion

Acquired aplastic anaemia, probably secondary to viral infection, is the most likely diagnosis. The blood film shows a pancytopenia with reduction in all three cell counts. Possible explanations for this are: (i) marrow failure, or (ii) hypersplenism leading to consumption of circulating cellular elements. The low reticulocyte count does not support the cause of red cell destruction being haemolysis by the spleen, as in this situation there should be an active marrow response; this therefore points to marrow failure. Marrow failure may be due to a genetic predisposition (e.g. Blackfan–Diamond syndrome, a pure red cell aplasia which occurs by 2 years of age in 95% of cases; Fanconi's anaemia; pancytopenia occurs in 25% of Schwachman–Diamond syndrome) or acquired. Many of the acquired aplastic anaemias are idiopathic but probably the commonest cause is after an acute viral (especially Epstein-Barr virus; parvovirus can produce red cell aplasia in patients with haemolytic anaemia but other cell lines can be affected) or bacterial infection. Other causes include drugs (e.g. chloramphenicol, nitrofurantoin, phenytoin, sulphonamides, carbimazole and cytotoxics), toxins (carbon tetrachloride, solvent abuse and insecticides) and radiation therapy. Rarer causes are autoimmune diseases and storage diseases. Malignant infiltration is excluded by the bone marrow biopsy.

The marrow in most cases of aplastic anaemia following viral infection will recover spontaneously and only supportive treatment with red cells, platelet transfusions and antibiotics is required in the interim period. If the cell counts fall to life-threatening levels, steroids may be given to stimulate the bone marrow and in a chronic unremitting aplastic anaemia, bone marrow transplantation may be considered.

Further reading
Milner A D, Hull D 1992 Hospital paediatrics, 2nd edn. Churchill Livingstone, Edinburgh, pp. 235 – 236

Answer 1.7

1. Venous stasis

Background

The first sample was difficult to take from the struggling child and the arm had been squeezed for several minutes causing venous stasis. Minimal venous stasis occurred when the senior house officer took blood.

If occlusion of vessels in the arm is maintained for more than a short time, water and small molecules pass from the lumen into surrounding interstitial fluid due to raised intravenous pressure and ischaemia of the vessel wall. Large molecules, such as proteins and red cell corpuscles, cannot pass through the vein wall at the same rate, resulting in a rise in their concentration.

Many plasma constituents are at least partly bound to protein. Prolonged venous stasis can thus raise the plasma calcium concentration as in this case. Prolonged stasis may also cause hypoxia with leakage of intracellular constituents, such as potassium and phosphate, causing falsely high plasma levels.

It is important to remember that concentrations of protein fractions and protein-bound substances may fall by as much as 15% after as little as 30 min of recumbency. Inpatients having blood taken early in the morning while recumbant tend to have lower values for protein fractions and protein-bound substances than outpatients.

Further reading

Zilva J F, Pannall P R, Mayne P D 1988 Clinical chemistry in diagnosis and treatment, 5th edn. Edward Arnold, London, pp. 477–448

Answer 1.8

1. Sarcoidosis
2. Kveim test
   Lymph node biopsy

Discussion

The diagnosis is suggested by the elevated angiotensin converting enzyme level, hilar lymphadenopathy and hypercalcaemia. Most cases of sarcoidosis in childhood are detected incidentally on chest X-ray, as in this child. The radiological changes in sarcoidosis are classified as follows:

Stage 1   Hilar node involvement
Stage 2   Diffuse mottling and strand-like opacities also seen
Stage 3   Some shrinkage of nodes and coalescent infiltrates
Stage 4   Emphysema, bullae, fibrosis and cor pulmonale

Monocytes, which are increased in sarcoidosis, are thought to be the cause of the raised angiotensin converting enzyme. The levels reflect disease activity and fall during remission. Elevated levels of angiotensin converting enzyme may also be found in other diseases such as leprosy and Gaucher's disease.

Hypercalcaemia is a recognized complication of sarcoidosis. Lung function tests may show a restrictive picture with impaired diffusing capacity.

A test that is often requested to aid diagnosis is the Kviem test. This is an intradermal injection of a homogenate from human sarcoid tissue. Four weeks later a nodular lesion with the histological features of sarcoidosis is produced in patients with sarcoidosis. The Kviem test, however, is often negative, especially in patients where sarcoidosis is confined to the lungs. Hence, the diagnosis often rests on the demonstration of sarcoid granulomata in tissue biopsy. Because of the high frequency of peripheral lymphadenopathy in childhood sarcoidosis, peripheral node biopsy is the most common source of material for biopsy. Lung biopsy is rarely necessary.

Further reading

Jasper P L, Denney F W 1968 Sarcoidosis in children with special emphasis on the natural history and treatment. Journal of Paediatrics 73: 499–512
Kendig E L 1974 The clinical picture of sarcoidosis in children. Pediatrics 24: 289–292
Lieberman J 1975 Elevation of serum angiotensin converting enzyme level in sarcoidosis. American Journal of Medicine 59: 356–372

Answer 1.9

1. Rickets
2. Bow legs
   Swollen wrists
   Pot belly
   Frontal skull bossing
   Rickety rosary
   Delayed closure of the anterior fontanelle (in younger children)

Discussion

The low plasma 25-hydroxycholecalciferol (HCC) and increased/normal parathyroid hormone suggest vitamin-D deficiency rickets (nutritional).

The biochemical results that help determine the cause of hypocalcaemia are:

	Calcium	Phosphate	Parathyroid hormone	Alkaline phosphatase
Hypoparathyroidsim	↓	↑	Low/undetectable	
Pseudohypoparathyroidism	↓	↑	↑	
Rickets	Normal/↓	↑ ↓		↑

Rickets can be classified by additional basal investigation:

Vitamin-D deficiency rickets (nutritional)	Plasma 25-HCC ↓ Parathyroid hormone ↑/normal
Vitamin-D dependent rickets type I	Plasma 25-HCC normal Plasma 1,25-DHCC ↓ Plasma parathyroid hormone ↑/normal
Vitamin-D dependent rickets type II (receptor defect)	Plasma 25-HCC normal Plasma 1,25-DHCC normal Plasma parathyroid hormone normal or ↑
Vitamin-D resistant (hypophophataemic) rickets	Plasma 25-HCC normal Plasma 1,25-DHCC normal Parathyroid hormone normal Phosphate ↓↓

Answer 1.10

1. Administration of insulin

Discussion

In this case, the mother, who was medically trained and diabetic, administered insulin injections to her child. This is a form of Munchausen by proxy syndrome. C-peptide is part of the connecting chain which remains intact during the conversion of pro-insulin to insulin. As it is excreted in equimolar amounts with insulin, it is a useful marker of β-cell function. Insulin and C-peptide measurements are independent of each other and are determined by radioimmunoassay. For example, it is possible to assess β-cell response to glucose in a diabetic patient receiving exogenous insulin. In the context of this patient with hypoglycaemic episodes, the C-peptide measurements can be valuable to document exogenous insulin administration.

Paper 2 *QUESTIONS*

Question 2.1

This is the audiogram from a $4\frac{1}{2}$-year-old girl who was referred because of severe speech delay.

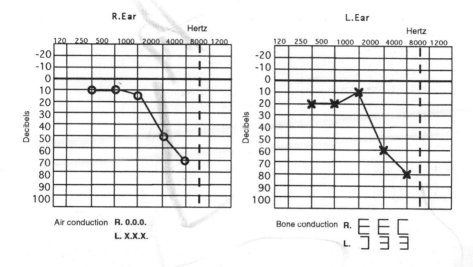

1. What does the audiogram show?
2. What is the cause of her speech delay?

Question 2.2

A 15-year-old boy had recurrent abdominal pain. This was not associated with vomiting. During an episode the following results were obtained:

Sodium	125 mmol/l
Plasma osmolality	260 mmol/kg
Urine osmolality	350 mmol/kg
Urinary porphobilinogen	Increased
Urinary 5-aminolaevulinate	Increased

There was no history of photosensitivity.

1. What is the most likely diagnosis?
2. What is the most likely cause of his hyponatraemia?

Question 2.3

This is the ECG trace from a 1-year-old girl following detection of a significant heart murmur. Clinically, she was thought to have a ventricular septal defect.

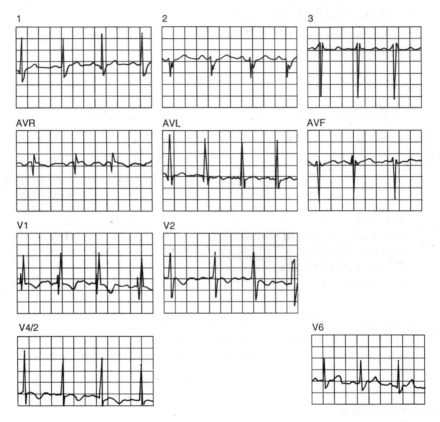

1. Give two significant abnormalities shown in the ECG.
2. What are the two most likely diagnoses?
3. In what syndrome does this condition commonly occur?

Question 2.4

An 8-year-old girl developed a pyrexia. She remained unwell and 3 days later developed pains in her limbs, particularly her thighs and upper arms. She subsequently complained of difficulty in breathing; her GP was called and she was referred to casualty. On examination she had flaccid weakness with absent reflexes. The power was greater in the right leg and the left arm and there was general weakness affecting the right side of the face with drooling. Sensory testing was equivocal. Lumbar puncture revealed the following results:

Lymphocytes 54/μl
Glucose   3.5 mmol/l
Protein   0.6 g/l

1. What is the most likely diagnosis?
2. Apart from examination and culture of the CSF, what three other investigations should be done?

Question 2.5

These results were obtained from a 3-month-old infant:

	Control	Baby	Baby following cryoprecipitate
Prothrombin ratio		3.5.	2.5
Activated partial prothrombin time (s)	46	144	142
Thrombin clotting time (TCT) (s)	16	23	20
TCT with protamine correction (s)	9	11	12
Reptilase time (s)	16	24	22

1. What is the haematological diagnosis?
2. What is the most likely underlying cause at this age?
3. Explain the effects of protamine correction on the TCT and reptilase time.

Question 2.6

A 1-year-old child is referred to you because the GP thinks he looks anaemic and bruises easily. Investigation shows the following results:

Blood:
Haemoglobin   7.0 g/dl
Platelet count   30 $\times$ 10^9/l
Ferritin   250 μg/l (normal 12–250 μg/l)
Urine:
Vanillylmandelic acid   50 μmol/mmol creatinine (upper limit of normal
                        15 μmol/mmol)
Homovanillic acid   55 μmol/mmol creatinine (upper limit of normal
                        25 μmol/mmol)

1. What is the likely diagnosis?

2. Suggest two other possible explanations for the urine results if the blood test had been normal.

Question 2.7

These are the different types of oesophageal atresia and tracheo-oesophageal fistulae.

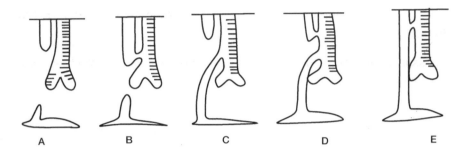

| A | B | C | D | E |

1. Which two types occur most commonly?
2. What radiological finding helps to differentiate between A and C in a newborn child?

Question 2.8

A 14-year-old child with sudden attacks of circumscribed, non-pitting, non-pruritic and painless oedema had the following laboratory results:

	During attacks	Between attacks
C2	Decreased	Normal
CH50	Decreased	
C3	Normal	Normal
C4	Decreased	Reduced
Haemolytic complement	Decreased	Reduced

1. What is the most likely diagnosis?
2. What test would help to confirm the diagnosis?

Question 2.9

A 5-year-old boy presented with short stature (−3.5 SD), his growth velocity was also <3rd centile. Following an insulin tolerance test, blood sugar dropped from 4.1 mmol/l to 1.7 mmol/l. Growth hormone increased from 1.4 mU/l to 3.5 mU/l. Growth hormone values were <0.5 mU/l throughout an arginine stimulation test.

1. What is the likely diagnosis?

Question 2.10

A 10-kg child presented with mild dehydration and a serum sodium of 120 mmol/l.

1. Assuming normal serum sodium is 135 mmol/l, what is the child's sodium deficit?

Paper 2 *ANSWERS*

Answer 2.1

1. Bilateral parital sensorineural deafness
2. Deafness

Discussion

The audiogram shows the recordings for air conduction only. However, it is clear that the loss is bilateral and in addition is confined to frequencies >1000 Hz. High-frequency loss is much more characteristic of sensorineural deafness than conductive deafness and therefore this diagnosis can be confidently made even in the absence of data on the bone conduction.

Loss of hearing frequencies >4000 Hz results in confusion of words with the same low-frequency component but different high-frequency components (e.g. 'feet' and 'seat' would both sound similar). Speech may be significantly improved by use of a hearing aid to boost these high frequencies. Speech delay suggests that the hearing loss is either longstanding or congenital. If it were a recent acute problem, speech would have developed and been acquired normally. Very high levels of neonatal jaundice can cause sensorineural deafness resulting in high frequency loss early in life.

Answer 2.2

1. Acute intermittent porphyria
2. Hypothalamic involvement producing inappropriate antidiuretic hormone secretion

Discussion

Acute intermittent porphyria is an autosomal dominant disorder associated with reduced activity of porphobilinogen D-aminase to approximately 50% of normal. It is one of the commonest forms of porphyria. The porphyrias are associated with defects in the biosynthesis of haem and over-production of haem precursors. Only approximately 10% of those who inherit the gene have clinical symptoms. Relatives should be screened for latent porphyria.

Symptoms usually begin after puberty and are more common in females than males. They are usually associated with an environmental precipitating factor. The acute intermittent attacks develop rapidly and then resolve over a period of days to weeks. They are characterized by the acute onset of severe abdominal pain followed by vomiting; pain and discomfort in the chest and extremities; urinary dysfunction; muscle weakness; mental disturbance such as anxiety, depression or disorientation; seizures; and occasionally bulbar and respiratory paralysis. Vomiting or inappropriate secretion of antidiuretic hormone may lead to hyponatraemia. Tachycardia and hypertension or hypotension may occur.

Clinical manifestations are due to a neuropathy, which involves anterior horn cells, dorsal root ganglion, splanchnic motor cells, cranial nerve nuclei and the hypothalamus. There is neuronal damage and axonal degeneration followed by demyelinization. Following a severe attack there may be residual weakness. Most patients are asymptomatic between attacks.

During attacks there is a marked increase in urinary excretion of ALA and PBG. The urine may turn brown or reddish on standing due to polymerization of PBG. Stool porphyrins are usually normal, which helps to differentiate acute intermittent porphyria from other forms that present with acute attacks. Once the disorder is clinically symptomatic, patients usually continue to excrete elevated ALA and PBG between acute attacks. The disorder may be confirmed by lowered activity of PBG deaminase in erythrocytes.

Treatment includes avoidance of hormones, drugs, alcohol, starvation and other factors known to be associated with acute attacks. During acute attacks, oral carbohydrate loading and intravenous glucose may be helpful. β-blockers may be needed to control tachycardia or hypertension.

Further reading

Campbell AGM, McIntosh N (eds) 1992 Forfar and Arneil's Textbook of paediatrics, 4th edn. Churchill Livingstone, Edinburgh, pp. 1209–1212
Hindmarsh J T 1986 The porphyrias: recent advances. Clinical Chemistry 45: 1255–1263

Answer 2.3

1. Left axis deviation
   Incomplete right bundle branch block
2. Ostium primum atrial septal defect
   Atrioventricular canal defect
3. Down's syndrome

Discussion

The ECG in both partial and complete atrioventricular septal defects characteristically shows these changes. A prolonged P-R interval is often seen. In ostium secundum atrial septal defects, the ECG shows right axis deviation and incomplete right bundle branch block.

The natural history of atrioventricular canal defects varies. In patients with an ostium primum atrial septal defect and minimal insufficiency of the left atrioventricular valve, the clinical course is similar to that of patients with a large ostium secundum atrial septal defect. These patients usually do well during childhood without treatment. During adulthood they have increasing tendency to develop congestive heart failure, particularly as atrial arrhythmias develop.

Patients with ostium primum atrial septal defects and moderate-to-severe left atrioventricular valve insufficiency will develop congestive cardiac failure early in life. Patients with complete atrioventricular canal defects develop severe symptoms with congestive cardiac failure in early infancy. They have frequent infections and fail to thrive. If they do survive infancy untreated, they generally develop pulmonary vascular disease.

Long-term results of surgical therapy depend on the degree of pre-operative pulmonary vascular disease and the extent of residual left atrioventricular valve regurgitation. Often the regurgitation is reduced substantially and the left-to-right shunt abolished by corrective surgery. When pulmonary vascular disease is present pre-operatively, mortality and morbidity rates are high. Post-operative arrhythmias can occur, including complete heart block, and may increase in incidence as patients grow older. With advancing age, mitral valve replacement may be required.

Further reading

Park M K, Guntheroff W G 1992 How to read pediatric ECGs, 2nd edn Mosby Yearbook, St Louis

Answer 2.4

1. Acute poliomyelitis

Guillain-Barré syndrome
Viral meningitis
2. Forced vital capacity
Throat swab for viral culture
Stool specimen for viral culture
Blood for viral titres

Discussion

The most likely diagnosis given the clinical information and CSF findings is acute poliomyelitis. This is now very rare in the UK but, although there are more common explanations for a fever followed by weakness, none fits with the data as well as polio. The particular clues are weakness that is asymmetrical and not confined to the limbs, in that there are respiratory symptoms, and unilateral nerve palsy; the CSF findings are typical of viral meningitis with a raised lymphocyte count, slightly raised protein and normal glucose.

The commonest cause in the UK of the onset of weakness and respiratory problems in a child following a febrile illness is Guillain-Barré syndrome (acute post-infective polyneuritis). Both acute poliomyelitis and Guillain-Barré syndrome can cause pains in the limbs and indeed this may be so severe in the latter that other symptoms are masked. Both disorders can also be associated with facial and bulbar palsies. Sensory abnormalities are never found in acute poliomyelitis but can occur in Guillain-Barré syndrome. However, sensory testing is notoriously difficult, particularly in children who are acutely ill and have difficulty concentrating. Therefore, the equivocal sensory findings should not lead to confusion in view of the CSF. In Guillain-Barré syndrome, the CSF may initially be normal during the first few days of symptoms, but if repeated again later in the illness will show a very raised CSF protein (up to 10–20 g/l), but with a normal cell count. The only other causes of such a high rise in the protein content of CSF are a complete block within the subarachnoid space (the usual cause is a spinal tumour, so-called Froin's syndrome) and neurofibromatosis (Von Recklinghausen's syndrome, an autosomal dominant disorder in which tumours arise from the peripheral nerves, nerve roots or cranial nerves, or sympathetic nervous tissue, giving rise to gliomas, meningiomas, acoustic neuromas, cutaneous fibromas and phaeochromocytoma).

Generalized weakness includes an enormous differential diagnosis which can be very confusing in the exam situation. The following classification may be helpful:

Spinal cord problem:	Trauma or atlanto-axial dislocation
	Bony abnormalities in Down's, achondroplasia or Morquio's syndrome
	Syringomyelia
	Tumour, e.g. dermoids, teratomas, gliomas, neuroblastomas, neurofibromas
	Abscess
	Post-infectious transverse myelitis
Anterior horn cell problem	Spinal muscular atrophy (Werdnig-Hoffman disease)
	Poliomyelitis
Motor nerve problem	
Focal neuropathy	Bell's palsy
	Brachial plexus injury at birth (Erb's palsy)
	Local trauma
Generalized motor neuropathy	Guillain-Barré syndrome
	Lead poisoning
	Acute intermittent porphyria
	Drugs, e.g. vincrisline
Neuromuscular junction	Myasesthenia gravis
Myopathy	Muscular dystrophy
	Dermatomyositis
	Mitochondrial myopathy
	Inhertited metabolic myopathies

Apart from CSF examination, the single most important test is to quantify the child's respiratory problems. In a child of 8 years, the forced vital capacity should be measured at least 4-hourly in the initial stages when paralysis may be advancing. If this is not available, crude alternatives are to ask the child to count out loud for as long as possible after a deep inspiration or to ask the child to cough. Non-invasive monitoring of oxygen saturation with pulse oximetry is helpful but tracheostomy and positive pressure ventilation should be instituted before hypoxia develops, as this may cause further neural damage and may be associated with pneumonia. Both acute poliomyelitis and Guillain-Barré syndrome may be associated with urinary retention due to bladder involvement. In the latter, autonomic involvement may also be associated with hypertension, whereas in polio, cardiac arrhythmias and heart failure can occur due to viral myocarditis.

The CSF should confirm the diagnosis microbiologically but the virus may also be recovered from throat swabs or stool cultures, and in addition acute and convalescent samples of serum should be taken 14 days apart to look for a rising antibody titre.

Acute poliomyelitis is rarely seen in the UK and occurs largely in non-immunized travellers from abroad or non-immunized siblings or parents of young children given live polio vaccine. Live polio vaccine can mutate on transmission through the gut into a more virulent form and the risk to household members in the UK is estimated at about 1 in 10^6 doses. For this reason oral polio vaccine is never given to infants on neonatal units until the moment of discharge. Many children infected with polio have a minor illness with gastroenteritis, fever and malaise. In a proportion, this progresses to a meningitic illness and in a proportion of these paralysis follows, which is then permanent, leading to the chronic features of weakness and muscle loss seen in survivors of polio.

Polio has largely been eradicated in the UK by the use of live Sabin vaccine, given in 3 doses at 2, 3 and 4 months of age. In other countries, a killed injectable (Salk) vaccine is used as there is greater certainty that the vaccine has been administered and less risk to non-immunized contacts. Killed vaccine is also recommended in children with immune deficiency who are at greater risk of paralytic polio. However, the Sabin type oral vaccine produces local IgA immunity in the gut, is easy and painless to administer and also induces a degree of herd immunity in the non-immunized through faecal secretion.

Further reading

Campbell AGM, McIntosh N (eds) 1992 Forfar and Arneil's Textbook of paediatrics, 4th edn. Churchill Livingstone, Edinburgh, pp. 1434–1437
Department of Health 1992 Immunisation against infectious disease. HMSO, London, pp. 50–52

Answer 2.5

1. Disseminated intravascular coagulation

2. Septicaemia

Shock
Major trauma
Extensive burns
Malignancy

3. If the prolonged TCT corrects with protamine, the prolongation is due to heparin or fibrin degradation products. The reptilase time is unaffected by heparin or fibrin degradation products

Discussion

The only haematological diagnosis that fits these data is disseminated intravascular coagulation. This laboratory diagnosis is based on a triad of thrombocytopenia, prolonged clotting times and elevated fibrin degradation products or a low fibrinogen level. This is because of simultaneous overactivity of both thrombosis and fibrinolysis with consumption of platelets and clotting factors. In addition, the widespread formation of fibrin plugs in the intravascular circulation may lead to a microangiopathic haemolytic anaemia with consumption of red cells. A degree of disseminated intravascular coagulation is more common as a laboratory finding than in clinical practice, when the diagnosis also requires there to be clinical evidence of overt bleeding or the formation of purpura or petechiae in the skin.

Septicaemia is the commonest cause of disseminated intravascular coagulation in children. In a term neonate, an alternative cause is birth asphyxia and in older children other causes include hypovolaemic shock, extensive trauma, burns and malignancy.

The commonest defects causing prolongation of activated partial thromboplastin time (APTT) are deficiencies of Factor VIII and IX (both sex-linked recessive disorders leading to haemophilia A and Christmas disease respectively). The commonest causes of prolongation of prothrombin time are a reduction in clotting factors II, VII, IX and X, all of which are vitamin-K dependent. Of these factors, Factor VII has the shortest half-life and therefore warfarin or acute liver disease will cause reduction in this factor first. Paradoxically, the prothrombin time is relatively insensitive to reduction in levels of prothrombin (Factor II).

TCT (also referred to as thrombin time) is the measure of haemostatically active fibrinogen and is prolonged by hypofibrinogenaemia, heparin and inhibitors of fibrin polymerization, such as the fibrin degradation products formed in disseminated intravascular coagulation. If the TCT corrects with the addition of protamine in the laboratory, then the originally prolonged TCT may have been due to either the presence of heparin or fibrin degradation products. However, if the reptilase time (which is unaffected by either heparin or fibrin degradation products) is prolonged, there is true hypofibrinogenaemia. This may have implications for therapy, as if the reptilase time is normal in the presence of clinical and laboratory diagnosis of disseminated intravascular coagulation, there is likely to be little clinical benefit from giving cryoprecipitate.

Treatment of disseminated intravascular coagulation remains controversial. Platelets and clotting factors should be given as sparingly as possible, as they simply fuel further consumption. However, if there is ongoing haemorrhage which is clinically significant and requires treatment, then platelets should be given and an attempt made to increase the circulating concentration of clotting factors. Human plasma protein fraction contains only 4% albumin and no clotting factors. Fresh frozen plasma contains all the clotting factors from blood donors but is not concentrated. However, fresh frozen plasma does include an a-II antiplasmin which inactivates the plasmin factor, which is increased in disseminated intravascular coagulation, and which causes the breakdown of fibrin to fibrin-degradation products. Cryoprecipitate, which is stored frozen and thawed before use, contains both Factor VIII (hence its use in haemophilia A but not haemophilia B) and fibrinogen. Fibrinogen is consumed in disseminated intravascular coagulation in the generation of fibrin plugs and this contributes to the secondary organ damage by interfering with tissue perfusion. The infant had a fibrinogen level of 0.6 g/l (normal range 2–4 g/l) and hence cryoprecipitate was given, but it can be seen from the data that this had only a marginal benefit on the prolonged clotting times.

Further reading

Wardle E N 1993 Coagulation problems in intensive care patients. Care of the Critically Ill 9: 246–249

Answer 2.6

1. Neuroblastoma
2. Muscular dystrophy
   Infected assay
   Stress response
   Phaeochromocytoma

Discussion

There is a low haemoglobin with a high ferritin — an extremely unusual combination, which is found in iron-loading disorders (e.g. haemosiderosis secondary to multiple transfusions in thalassaemia and sideroblastic anaemias). However, the combination of thrombocytopenia with anaemia suggests a differential diagnosis of hypersplenism, disseminated intravascular coagulation, haemolytic uraemic syndrome or marrow infiltration. The only one of these associated with a high ferritin is neuroblastoma leading to infiltration of the marrow. This diagnosis is confirmed by the increased urinary catecholamines.

Neuroblastoma accounts for about 7% of all childhood malignancies, most occurring in the first 5 years of life and three-quarters presenting as an abdominal mass, although the tumour may arise in any of the tissues of the sympathetic nervous system. Because of early dissemination and the possibility that the primary may be in any tissue derived from neural crest cells, there are many different clinical manifestations of neuroblastoma; the most common primary site is the adrenal gland.

Apart from presenting as an abdominal mass, or as with any other disseminated tumour, with failure to thrive or features of marrow infiltration, this malignancy can also present with neurological signs. Local infiltration can produce spinal extradural tumours and enlargement of an intravertebral foramen is sometimes seen on plain X-rays of the spine. Cervical disease can produce Horner's syndrome. A syndrome of acute cerebellar ataxia and rapid eye movements may rarely be seen at presentation. The differential diagnosis of this is ataxia telangiectasia which may be complicated by a lymphoma.

Ninety per cent of neuroblastomas are associated with raised levels of one or both of vanillylmandelic acid and homovanillic acid, which are catecholamine metabolites. Although catecholamine levels may be very high, they do not usually cause hypertension, which is more typically seen in nephroblastoma (two-thirds of which occur before the age of 3 years, and account for 5% of all childhood malignancies) and the much rarer phaeochromocytoma. Ferritin is produced in neuroblastoma cells and is elevated in about half the cases of advanced stage disease. The levels of catecholamines are also raised in blood but urinary assay is easier and initially a spot urine sample is adequate. If any doubt remains about the diagnosis, a 24-h urine collection should be made but this is more difficult. The absolute concentrations are not a guide to prognosis but serial measurements can be used to monitor the effectiveness of treatment.

False positive results may arise either because the urine concentration of creatinine is abnormally low (e.g. in muscular dystrophy or if the urine is collected on filter paper which then becomes infected leading to preferential consumption of creatinine by the bacteria), or because of high concentrations of homovanillic acid or vanillylmandelic acid, reflecting high circulating catecholamine levels as a stress response to a serious illness (e.g. congenital heart disease, failure to thrive, pneumonia). However, false positives usually give rise to only a modest elevation in the catecholamine metabolites, whereas concentrations over 100 μmol/mmol creatinine strongly suggest a true positive case.

The final cause of raised urinary catecholamine metabolites is a phaeochromocytoma. These arise from the chromaffin cells and therefore, like neuroblastoma, can arise from anywhere in the sympathetic chain in the abdomen, the mediastinum, the neck or from the adrenal medulla (two-thirds of cases). It may be sporadic or familial in association with the autosomal dominant multiple endocrine neoplasia syndromes or with neurofibromatosis. They may present with either paroxysomal or sustained hypertension, leading to severe headaches or hypertensive cardiac failure. Other catecholamine symptoms such as sweating, nausea and vomiting may be seen. They do not present with features of bone marrow failure.

Further reading

Campbell AGM, McIntosh N (eds) 1992 Forfar and Arneil's Textbook of paediatrics, 4th edn. Churchill Livingstone, Edinburgh, pp. 984–987

Parker L, Craft A W, Dale G et al 1992 Screening for neuroblastoma in the north of England. British Medical Journal 305: 1260–1263

Answer 2.7

1. C and A   *NO*
2. Only in A will there be gas in the stomach

Discussion

The frequences of the different types are C (85%), A (9%), E (4%), B (1%) and D (1%). In patients with the defect shown in A, there is no connection between oesophagus, trachea or stomach. Hence, no gas is found in the stomach. The presence of air in the stomach is proof of a fistula between the distal oesophagus and trachea. *only at birth, otherwise, swallowed air ē feed*

In newborns suspected of oesophageal atresia, an attempt should be made to pass a large, flexible catheter into the stomach. The catheter will be felt to stick at about 8–10 cm. The position of the obstruction is confirmed by chest and abdomen X-rays. *(6% False -ve; H Type, prox. connection)*

Following the operative repair of oesophageal atresia, respiratory problems are common. In the first 5 years, 20% have radiological evidence of pneumonia, 40% wheeze and 80% bronchitis. 75% have a persistent harsh cough during the early years — the so-called TOF cough. Respiratory problems become less frequent after the age of 5 years.

TOF via proximal end of oesoph only: 1%, db cases
TOF ~ distal ~ ~ ~ only: 85% ~ ~

Further reading

Chetcuti P, Phelan P D 1993 Respiratory morbidity after repair of oesophageal atresia and tracheo-oesophageal fistula. Archives of Disease in Childhood 68: 167–170

Answer 2.8

1. Recurrent angioedema due to C1 esterase inhibitor deficiency
2. Measurement of C1 esterase inhibitor

Discussion

Recurrent angioedema may be associated with hereditary C1 esterase deficiency and usually has autosomal dominant inheritance. Triggers include trauma, emotional upset, infection and menses. In children, a rash resembling erythema marginatum may also spread with the swelling. Angioedema may be life threatening if it involves the airway. Attacks are uncommon in early childhood and often worsen after puberty.

About 15% of all patients with hereditary angioneurotic oedema have a biologically inactive form of C1 esterase inhibitor, which is immunochemically identical with normal. Thus, in patients with normal C1 esterase inhibitor levels and a typical history, a functional assay of C1 esterase inhibitor is required.

Because inheritance is autosomal dominant, C1 esterase inhibitor is not usually completely absent but is severely depleted during an acute attack. Anabolic steroids such as danazol increase C1 esterase inhibitor production and are useful in treatment. Tranexamic acid inhibits plasmin, which activates and consumes C1 esterase inhibitor. Given in combination these drugs have proved beneficial.

Further reading

Watson J G, Bird A G 1989 Handbook of immunological investigations in children. Wright, Bristol, pp. 116–118

Answer 2.9

1. Isolated growth hormone deficiency

Discussion

It is now recommended that the insulin tolerance test is avoided whenever possible and, if it must be done, is conducted only in a specialist centre. Blood glucose must be monitored frequently. Insulin-induced hypoglycaemia acts as a stimulus for growth hormone release and during the test symptoms of hypoglycaemia usually occur within 30 min of insulin injection. The blood glucose should decrease by 50% or more of the basal value and there should be symptoms and signs of hypoglycaemia: drowsiness, sweating, headache and occasionally nausea and vomiting. With adequate hypoglycaemia, peak growth hormone levels of <7 mU/l indicate growth hormone deficiency and this is excluded with levels >15 mU/l. Intermediate levels may indicate partial growth hormone deficiency requiring confirmation with a second, but different, test for growth hormone secretion.

Arginine was used in this patient as a second test of growth hormone secretion. It is infused intravenously over a 30-min period, and blood collected for growth hormone over 90 min. The interpretation of growth hormone levels is similar to that during the insulin tolerance test. Growth hormone response to profound hypoglycaemia in this patient was minimal. The deficiency was confirmed when growth hormone levels were almost undetectable following arginine stimulation.

Further reading
Campbell AGM, McIntosh N (eds) Forfar and Arneil's Textbook of paediatrics, 4th edn. Churchill Livingstone, Edinburgh, pp. 1089–92

Answer 2.10

1. 90 mmol

Discussion

Serum sodium levels can be used to calculate the approximate amount of sodium required to correct any deficit. Sodium is distributed through a volume greater than the extracellular fluid. In fact, the total exchangeable pool of sodium is about 0.6 l/kg (60%) of body weight. The amount of sodium required to restore the plasma concentration to normal (135 mmol/l) in a depleted patient can be calculated from the equations:

Sodium deficit (mmol) = (135 − observed sodium concentration) × 0.6 × body weight

where:

Sodium distribution volume (l) = 0.6 × body weight (kg)

This child has dehydration, so the low serum sodium reflects a sodium deficit rather than haemodilution from over-hydration. The sodium deficit per litre of plasma is 135 − 120 = 15 mmol/l. Sodium is distributed through a volume of 0.6 × 10 = 6 litres. Therefore, the total serum deficit is 15 × 6 = 90 mmol.

Paper 3 QUESTIONS

Question 3.1

This audiogram is from a 6-year-old boy who was referred because he was not doing well at school. There had been no other symptoms. A hearing test 2 months before showed similar findings.

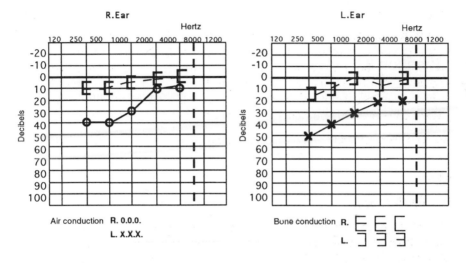

Air conduction R. 0.0.0.
L. X.X.X.

Bone conduction R. ⊏ ⊏ ⊏
L. ⅃ ⅃ ⅃

1. What does the audiogram show?
2. What is the likely pathology?
3. What two things should you do?

Question 3.2

An ECG trace (A) was taken from an unconscious 10-year-old child who had been rescued from the North Sea. The child's condition deteriorated and a second ECG strip was obtained (B).

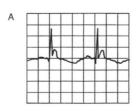

A

B

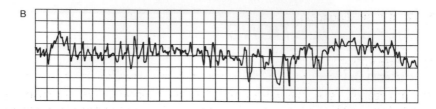

1. What does ECG trace A show?
2. What does ECG trace B show?

Question 3.3

These are the results from a cardiac catheterization performed on an infant with an ejection systolic murmur and a history of recurrent chest infections.

	Oxygen saturation (%)	Blood pressure (mmHg) (systolic/diastolic)
Right atrium	87	—/6
Right ventricle	86	35/5
Pulmonary artery	86	35/15
Left atrium	96	—/6
Left ventricle	96	—
Aorta	96	—

1. What is the most likely diagnosis?
2. Give three ECG abnormalities that may be seen in such cases.

Question 3.4

A 10-month-old boy presented with purpura and a large haemangioma of the left hand and forearm.

Haemoglobin	9 g/dl
Platelet count	18×10^9/l
Prothrombin time	Normal
Partial thromboplastin time	Normal
Thrombin time	Normal
Fibrinogen	0.5 g/l

1. What is the diagnosis?

Question 3.5

You are called to see an 8-year-old child whose conscious level is continuing to deteriorate 48 h after he has had lumbar puncture for headaches and fever. He has been treated for a further 48 h with intravenous benzyl penicillin and cefotaxime. The CSF findings are:

Lymphocytes	98/mm^3
Polymorphs	76/mm^3
Gram stain	No organisms seen
Protein	1.1 g/l
CSF glucose	0.5 mmol/l
Blood glucose	5.6 mmol/l

1. What is the most likely explanation for the failure of antibiotic therapy?
2. Suggest three tests that might confirm this diagnosis?

Question 3.6

A 10-year-old Asian girl is investigated because her parents are concerned about her poor appetite. The history is otherwise unremarkable and there are no other gastrointestinal symptoms. The girl was born in the UK following a healthy pregnancy and normal delivery but the parents recall that she was jaundiced after birth, although this did not require any specific treatment. Examination is unremarkable and a blood test shows the following results:

Haemoglobin	9.5 g/dl
Mean corpuscular volume	71 fl
HbA$_2$	2%
Blood film	Hypochromic red cells

The father knows he has β-thalassaemia trait.

1. Can you reassure the parents that their daughter does not have β-thalassaemia minor or major?

Question 3.7

An 8-year-old girl presented with epistaxes. The following laboratory results were obtained:

Full blood count	Microcytic hypochromic anaemia
Platelet count	Normal
Haemoglobin	9 g/dl
MCV	60 fl
Red blood cells	Hypochromic
Prothrombin time	Normal
Partial thromboplastin time	56 s (control 42 s)
Thrombin time	Normal
Factor VIII:C	25%
Factor VIIIR:Ag	27%
Bleeding time	13 min (control 6 min)
Platelet retention to glass	Reduced
Platelet aggregation to ristocetin	Reduced

1. What is the most likely diagnosis?
2. What is the mode of inheritance?

Question 3.8

This is the trace of the lung volumes measured by a spirometer.

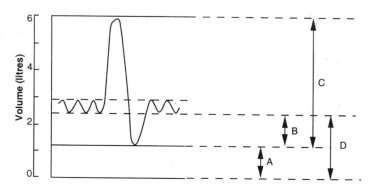

1. What do the letters represent?
2. What will happen to 'D' in a patient during a significant asthmatic attack?

Question 3.9

An obese 2-year-old girl was found to be hypocalcaemic and did not respond to vitamin D. These results were found:

Plasma calcium	1.2 mmol/l
Plasma phosphate	2.8 mmol/l (normal 0.8–1.4 mmol/l)

Alkaline phosphatase	300 IU/l
Urea	4 mmol/l
Albumin	39 g/l
Magnesium	0.7 mmol/l
Parathyroid hormone	20 ng/ml (normal <1.0 ng/ml)

1. What is the most likely diagnosis?
2. What may radiological examination of the hand reveal?
3. How may the response to parathyroid hormone infusion confirm the diagnosis?

Question 3.10

These are the results from a healthy 14-year-old boy known to have hyperlipidaemia:

Sodium	122 mmol/l
Plasma osmolarity	270 mmol/l
Plasma osmolality	289 mmol/kg

1. What is the most likely explanation of the low serum sodium measurement?
2. How do you explain the difference between the plasma osmolality and osmolarity?

Paper 3 *ANSWERS*

Answer 3.1

1. Bilateral conductive deafness
2. Bilateral serous otitis media

   Bilateral glue ear

3. Refer to an ENT surgeon
   Inform the school teacher
   Trial of treatment with an antibiotic *and* either an antihistamine or a decongestant such as ephedrine

   Trial of treatment with an antihistamine
   Trial of treatment with a decongestant

   (Tympanometry would be a poor answer as the diagnosis can be made from the audiogram)

Discussion

The audiogram shows a bilateral deficit which involves loss of air conduction but little loss of bone conduction. The loss of air conduction is greatest at low frequencies, which is characteristic of a conductive loss rather than a sensorineural loss. The deficit is mild, which again favours a conductive loss. As a rough rule of thumb, losses of up to 20 dcb cause little or no problem with hearing or normal conversation, losses of 20–40 dcb result in difficulty hearing normal conversation, which would be heard as a whisper, losses of 40–60 dcb result in difficulty hearing loud speech such as a teacher's voice, and losses of 60–80 dcb involve difficulty in hearing a very loud voice or shout, which would probably not be understood at all. The commonest caues of bilateral hearing loss in a school-age child is secretory otitis media.

   One pragmatic approach to management would be to try a 6-week course of decongestants (ephedrine and antihistamine) and an antibiotic, and then to repeat the audiogram. If there is no improvement, referral to an ENT surgeon for consideration of insertion of grommets would be reasonable. Chronic and fluctuating conductive hearing loss can greatly impair school performance and it is vital that the child's teacher is informed of the problem, so that the child can be seated at the front of the class.

Answer 3.2

1. J-wave (Osborne wave)
2. Ventricular fibrillation

Discussion

The J-wave is a hump-like wave superimposed on the distal limb of the QRS complex, which may be seen in patients with hypothermia. Hypothermia also causes prolongation of the Q–T interval, sinus bradycardia and often shivering artefact.

Ventricular fibrillation is characterized by a bizarre ventricular QRS pattern of varying size and configuration. The rate is rapid and irregular. This is a terminal arrhythmia as it cannot provide effective perfusion of the myocardium. Successful resuscitation depends upon prompt recognition.

Further reading

Park M K, Gunteroff W G 1992 How to interpret pediatric ECGs, 2nd edn. Mosby Yearbook, St Louis

Answer 3.3

1. Secundum atrial septal defect
2. Incomplete right bundle branch block
   Right axis deviation (or normal axis)
   Right atrial and right ventricle hypertrophy
   First-degree heart block

Discussion

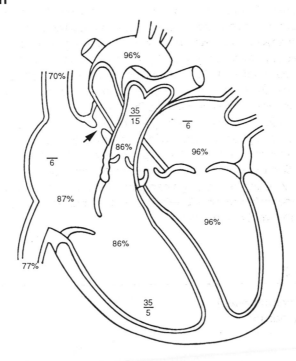

The most likely diagnosis is an atrial septal defect. Partial anomalous pulmonary venous drainage may also cause a rise in blood oxygen saturation in the right atrium but is less common. Children with an atrial septal defect are usually asymptomatic. An increased frequency of respiratory tract infections and mild exercise intolerance may occur. Heart failure can occasionally develop in infants with large defects.

The chest X-ray may show cardiomegaly with enlargement of the right atrium and increased pulmonary vascularity. Cross-sectional echocardiography will reveal the site and size of the defect. This is usually sufficient to provide the diagnosis in children and cardiac catheterization is not required before surgery. Surgery is usually recommended between the age of 2 and 5 years.

Further reading

Campbell A G M, McIntosh N (eds) 1992 Forfar and Arneil's Textbook of paediatrics, 4th edn. Churchill Livingstone, Edinburgh, pp. 674–675

Answer 3.4

1. Kasabach–Merritt syndrome

Discussion

The association of giant cavernous haemangiomas and thrombocytopenia is referred to as Kasabach–Merritt syndrome. The thrombocytopaenia is usually caused by intravascular coagulation localized to the haemangioma and thrombi do not occur at other sites. Consumptive coagulopathy within haemangioma may be enough to consume platelets and coagulation factors below haemostatic levels, resulting in bleeding manifestations at other distant sites. Fibrinogen levels may be particularly low. Patients have developed thrombocytopenia with lesions as small as 6 cm, although haemangiomas leading to the Kasabach–Merritt syndrome are usually considerably larger.

Answer 3.6

1. Tuberculous meningitis

Bacterial meningitis with resistant organism
Cerebral abscess

2. Ziehl–Neilson stain of cerebrospinal fluid
CSF culture for mycobacterium tuberculosis

Mantoux test

Chest X-ray
CT brain scan

Discussion

This child has CSF containing raised numbers of both lymphocytes and polymorphs (beyond the newborn period the maximum number of lymphocytes/mm^3 is 5 and there should be no polymorphs at all), but apparently no organisms. In addition, the protein is raised (upper limit of normal range is 0.15–0.45 g/l) and the glucose is extremely low (anything <60% of a simultaneous blood glucose is abnormal and, irrespective of the blood glucose, a CSF glucose of 0.5 mmol/l is clearly very low). There are a number of possibilities to differentiate.

If the child had already received antibiotics prior to lumbar puncture, then a mixed pleocytosis may be seen in the absence of organisms. However, CSF glucose would not normally be this low. In an 8-year-old child the most likely organisms are meningococcus and pneumococcus. Haemophilus meningitis is not often seen beyond the age of 5 years and viral meningitis does not explain the very low CSF sugar. All three of these bacterial organisms are sensitive to the combination of benzyl penicillin and cefotaxime and the child would not be expected to continue to deteriorate once antibiotics had been started, particularly given early in the illness prior to lumbar puncture. There is recent evidence that children given intramuscular penicillin by their GP before referral to hospital with meningococcal disease have a better outcome than those in whom antibiotics have been deferred until after lumbar puncture.

The second possibility is that the child has a cerebral abscess. This can cause meningeal irritation, explaining the headaches and the pleocytosis and raised protein in the CSF, but whilst the organisms remain confined to the abscess, the CSF will be sterile. If the abscess is causing a space-occupying mass effect, then the child will continue to deteriorate despite the intravenous broad-spectrum antibiotics and the correct management here is CT scan to localize the abscess and neurosurgical drainage of the abscess under general anaesthesia. Again, however, pyogenic abscess would not be expected to cause such a low CSF glucose and therefore the answer would receive fewer marks than the best answer which is tuberculous meningitis.

Tuberculous meningitis explains the CSF findings and the lack of response to broad-spectrum intravenous antibiotics. Tuberculous meningitis and an intracranial abscess may be difficult to distinguish. Both may present with an indolent history of several weeks of headache, fever and rather non-specific symptoms, rather than classical acute menigism, and both may be associated with papilloedema. Bacterial menigitis very rarely causes papilloedema even when there is raised intracranial pressure as the onset is rapid, but papilloedema is well recognized in tuberculous meningitis which has a more gradual onset.

The Ziehl-Neilson stain tests for acid-fast bacilli. The more CSF obtained at lumbar puncture and the more times the microbiologist looks, the more likely the organism is to be found (the success rate varies from 30% to 90% in different centres). CSF should also be cultured for at least 6 weeks on Lowenstein–Jensen medium as this is essential for the isolation of tubercle bacilli present in small numbers and to assess drug resistance.

If the microbiological diagnosis cannot be made from microscopy or culture, the diagnosis can be confirmed by a Mantoux test. A 25 gauge needle is used to inject 0.1 ml of tuberculin-purified protein derivative solution intradermally on the upper third of the flexor aspect of the forearm and the skin is assessed at 48 and 72 h. The test is regarded as positive if there is a reaction consisting of a raised area of inflammatory oedema (i.e. 'induration') not <5 mm in diameter, and negative if there is 0–4 mm induration or immediate non-specific reaction which completely disappears by 48 h. A routine test is carried out with a 1 in 1000 tuberculin-purified protein derivative. If tuberculosis is strongly suspected, or the patient is known to be hypersensitive to tuberculin, the more dilute 1 in 10 000 derivative should be used initially. If there is no reaction and there is a strong clinical suspicion of tuberculosis, then it should be repeated with 1 in 1000 tuberculin. However, it should be remembered that a positive Mantoux test may occur because a child has previously had a BCG immunization.

Answers receiving fewer marks are chest X-ray (looking for evidence of tuberculosis) and CT brain scan (to exclude an abscess).

In the UK, tuberculous menigitis is a rare diagnosis but is easily missed if not suspected. It is commonest in children under 5 years and those whose families come from the Asian subcontinent. Even if Asian children are born in the UK and never travel back to the Asian subcontinent, they remain a high-risk group because they are frequently in contact with relatives who may have tuberculosis.

Further reading

Campbell A G M, McIntosh N (eds) 1992 Forfar and Arneil's Textbook of paediatrics, 4th edn. Churchill Livingstone, Edinburgh, pp. 1400–1401
Department of Health 1992 Immunisation against infections disease. HMSO, London, p. 14, 82

Answer 3.6

1. No

Discussion

You can reassure the parents that their daughter is not homozygous for β-thalassaemia major, but she may be a carrier of the β-thalassaemia minor trait like her father. The β-thalassaemias arise due to lack of one or both of the genes necessary for synthesis of the β-chain of the globin polypeptide. Normal adult haemoglobin, HbA, which accounts for over 90% of the haemoglobin in healthy normal children beyond the first 3 months of age, is made up of two α- and two β-chains. Haemoglobin F has a high affinity for oxygen and is therefore useful in fetal life, accounting for three-quarters of the haemoglobin at the time of birth. However, HbF levels fall to <2% by the first year of life. In β-thalassaemia, β-chains cannot be produced and a compensatory response in postnatal life to maintain the haemoglobin concentration is to produce more HbA_2 (two α chains and two δ chains) or more HbF (two α chains and two γ chains). As a result, the usual picture in the homozygous β-thalassaemic is for HbF to be raised to between 10% and 90% and HbA_2 to be raised to 10%. In β-thalassaemia minor, both HbF and HbA_2 are raised to between 3% and 10%.

However, a common source of confusion in β-thalassaemia minor is the concomitant presence of iron-deficiency anaemia. Both β-thalassaemia and iron deficiency are accompanied by microcytosis, but the latter tends to cause a reduction of HbA_2 levels, whereas in the former it may be normal, as in this case, and haemoglobin electrophoresis should be repeated once the iron deficiency has been corrected. Iron-deficiency anaemia is common in the Asian population, because of late weaning and dietary mores. Many Hindu families are vegetarian.

The best test to ensure that this child does not have this combination is a serum ferritin concentration, which will be low in iron-deficiency anaemia, but normal in β-thalassaemia minor and major. Serum ferritin is a more useful indicator than serum iron, as the latter is more vulnerable to fluctuations of dietary intake and concurrent illness. Serum ferritin is a measure of the total iron stored within the body and the normal range is age-dependent. At birth dietary iron stores are high to cope with the fact that breast milk is a relatively poor source of iron (1 mg/l). Antepartum haemorrhage or postnatal blood loss will deplete the body stores of iron, particularly in a preterm infant. Iron stores fall over the first 6 months of life and then remain stable throughout childhood on a normal mixed diet without supplementation. The dietary requirements of a normal infant are about 1 mg/kg/day but only 10% of this is absorbed across the gastrointestinal tract. Iron-deficiency anaemia can be corrected with a 3-month course of oral iron equivalent to 2 mg/kg/day. The parents and child should be warned that this will make the stools appear dark (which may be confused with melaena, particularly if the cause of the iron-deficiency anaemia has been gastrointestinal blood loss) and may lead to either constipation or loose stools, and sometimes abdominal pain. As a result of these side effects, despite anticipatory warnings, compliance is often poor and the ferritin should be repeated at 3 months to check for a good therapeutic effect. If iron has been taken until symptoms of tiredness resolve and appetite and temperament improve, and then discontinued, the blood film and serum iron at 3 months may be normal but the serum ferritin will remain low. This is because the iron stores have not been adequately replenished and a further 3-month course should be prescribed with the emphasis on compliance.

Answer 3.7

1. Classical Von Willebrand's disease (Type 1)
2. Autosomal dominant

Discussion

Von Willebrand's disease involves primary defects or deficiencies in the Von Willebrand portion of the Factor VIII complex, with variable deficiencies of Factor VIII:C, the pro-coagulant component of the Factor VIII molecule. Abnormalities of Von Willebrand factor result in increased platelet adhesiveness, impairment of agglutination of platelets in the presence of ristocetin, and prolongation of the bleeding time.

There are two major forms of Von Willebrand's disease, quantitative or qualitative. Mild quantitative abnormalities are referred to as Type 1 Von Willebrand's disease. Qualitative abnormalities are termed Type 2. Clinically, patients show a mild-to-moderate bleeding tendency, usually involving the mucocutaneous surfaces. Epistaxis, haemorrhage after dental extraction and increased bruising are common problems. Menorrhagia and melaena may occur.

Treatment of Type I Von Willebrand's disease is usually with DDAVP (desamino D-arginine vasopressin). The effect of DDAVP on bleeding time lasts approximately 3−4 h. Cryoprecipitate contains intact Von Willebrand's factor and is effective in treating all subtypes.

	VIII:C (coagulant)	VIIIR:Ag (related antigen)	VIIIR:Wf (Von Willebrand factor)
Classical haemophilia	+++	Normal	Normal
Haemophilia carrier	+ (e.g. 50%)	Normal	Normal
Von Willebrand's	++ (e.g. 25%)	++	++

In contrast to haemophilia A, Von Willebrand's disease is usually transmitted as an autosomal dominant trait. Homozygous cases do occur and are severely affected.

Further reading

Milner A D, Hull D 1992 Hospital paediatrics, 2nd edn. Churchill Livingstone, Edinburgh, pp. 237−240

Answer 3.8

1. A = residual lung volume
   B = expiratory reserve volume

C = vital capacity

D = functional residual capacity

2. Increase

Discussion

Each subdivision is called a 'volume' while any combination of two or more volumes is called a 'capacity'. Total lung capacity (TLC) is the volume of gas in the lungs and airways after a maximal inspiration. The residual volume (RV) is the volume of air in the lungs and airways after a maximal expiration. Vital capacity is the volume of the deepest possible breath from maximal inspiration to maximal expiration (TLC−RV). Functional residual capacity is the volume of gas in the lungs at the end of a normal expiration. Tidal volume is the volume of a particular breath. *at rest*

During an asthmatic attack, air trapping occurs and the patient becomes hyperinflated. Functional residual capacity is therefore increased.

Further reading

West J B 1989 Respiratory physiology: the essentials, 4th edn. Williams & Wilkins, Baltimore

Answer 3.9

1. Pseudohypoparathyroidism

2. Short 4th metacarpal

3. No urinary phosphate, cAMP or plasma calcium response

Discussion

Pseudohypoparathyroidism is due to the failure of response of the renal tubules to parathormone stimulation. It seems to be transmitted as an incompletely penetrant dominant gene. The condition occurs more frequently in females and onset is during childhood. Presenting symptoms are recurring tetany and convulsions, muscle cramps, paraesthesiae and stridor. Mental retardation, growth failure, cataracts and calcification of the basal ganglia may occur.

Whilst the above features may also be common to true hypoparathyroidism, the occurence of subcutaneous calcification and shortening of the metacarpal bones is confined to pseudohypoparathyroidism.

The elevated parathyroid hormone and the presence of hypocalcaemia suggest the diagnosis. Renal response to parathyroid hormone infusion is a dynamic investigation to determine the cause of hypoparathyroidism. The response is measured by urinary phosphate and cAMP response to parathyroid hormone. In patients with pseudohypoparathyroidism, there is no response. In patients with hypoparathyroidism there is marked increase in plasma and urinary cAMP and an increase in urinary phosphate excretion. Plasma calcium may also be increased.

Further reading

Campbell A G M, McIntosh N (eds) 1992 Forfar and Arneil's Textbook of paediatrics, 4th edn. Churchill Livingstone, Edinburgh, pp. 1027–1028, 1129–1130

Answer 3.10

2 *. Lipaemia may cause measured sodium levels and calculated osmolarity to be significantly lower than their true concentrations in plasma water *(osmolality*

1 *. The apparent hyponatremia is due to the patient's hyperlipaemia

Discussion

Osmolar concentrations can be expressed as osmolarity (mmol/l of solution) or osmolality (mmol/kg of solvent). Under normal conditions, although measured osmolality should be higher than calculated osmolarity (because this calculation omits the protein in the plasma), there is little difference between the two. Osmolarity can be calculated, e.g.:

$$2(Na^+) + 2(K^+) + (urea) + (glucose)$$

This is usually adequate for clinical purposes. However, the relationship does not hold in gross hyperlipidaemia or hyperproteinaemia. In the case of this boy, the lipid contributes much more than the 6% occupied by plasma proteins.

Further reading

Zilva J F, Pannall P R, Mayne P D 1988 Clinical chemistry in diagnosis and treatment, 5th edn. Edward Arnold, London

Paper 4 *QUESTIONS*

Question 4.1

Two children attending the neurology clinic were discovered to have visual field defects.

  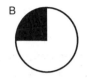

1. Damage to what part of the visual pathway would produce the visual field effects seen in A?
2. Damage to what part of the visual pathway would produce the visual field effects seen in B?

Question 4.2

This is the ECG trace from a 6-year-old boy.

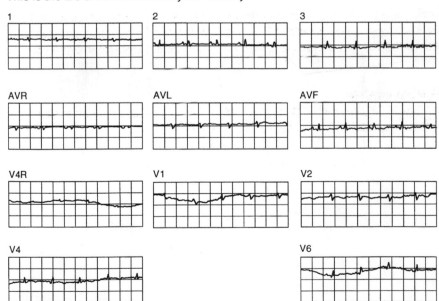

1. Why is this ECG trace abnormal?
2. Give six causes of this ECG appearance.

Question 4.3

These are the cardiac catheter findings from a 1-year-old boy with a heart murmur.

	Oxygen saturation (%)	Blood pressure (mmHg) (systolic/diastolic)
Right atrium	75	—
Right ventricle	75	38/5
Pulmonary artery	85	38/15
Left atrium	96	—
Left ventricle	96	—
Aorta	96	110/60

1. What is the diagosis?
2. What abnormalities may be found on his ECG?

Question 4.4

Prenatal ultrasound scanning at 20 weeks gestation identified a cardiac abnormality in the developing fetus. This was the first pregnancy to a healthy, unrelated couple, both in their twenties. Urgent amniocentesis and chromosome analysis yielded the karyotype shown.

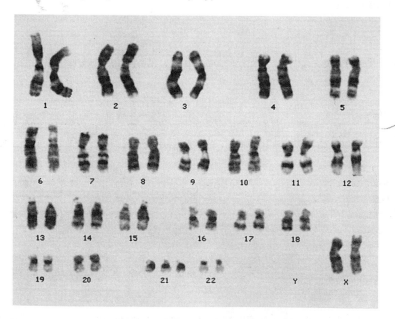

1. What is the diagnosis?
2. What might the maternal serum α-fetoprotein have shown?

3. What is the approximate incidence of the condition given the parents' ages?
4. What level of reoccurrence may be expected?

Question 4.5

A 4-year-old boy with non-Hodgkin's lymphoma presents with a 24-h history of headache and a 'flu-like' illness. Lumbar puncture gave the following results:

White cell count $720 \times 10^6/l$
Polymorphonuclear
   leucocytes   70%
Red cell count $20 \times 10^6/l$
CSF glucose   2.5 mmol/l
Plasma glucose   6.0 mmol/l
Protein   1.9 g/l
Gram stain   Occasional Gram-positive bacilli, reported by
                       telephone as contaminating diptheroids
Full blood count:
Haemoglobin   12.2 g/dl
White cell count $9.1 \times 10^9/l$
Neutrophils   90%
Red cell count $4.51 \times 10^{12}/l$
Platelet count $261 \times 10^9/l$

1. What is the likely diagnosis?
2. What is the treatment of choice if this diagnosis is confirmed?

Question 4.6

These are the results of a full blood count from a 6-year-old boy.

Haemoglobin   9.2 g/dl
Mean corpuscular volume   82 fl
White cell count $8 \times 10^9/l$
Platelet count $235 \times 10^9/l$

The blood film was reported as showing two populations of red cells of different sizes.

1. Suggest four possible explanations for this blood result.
2. Give the four best investigations which would help differentiate between these.

Question 4.7

A 3-year-old caucasian child presents with fever, diarrhoea and vomiting. Investigation shows the following blood test results:

Plasma potassium	2.8 mmol/l
Plasma sodium	135 mmol/l
Plasma urea	8.3 mmol/l
Haemoglobin	8.4 g/dl
Blood film	Polychromasia, schistocytes and toxic granulation
White cell count	12×10^9/l
Platelet count	36×10^9/l
Activated partial prothrombin time	40 s (38 s in control)
Prothrombin ratio	1.1

1. What type of anaemia is this?
2. Give three simple tests which would help support this?
3. What is the most likely underlying diagnosis?

Question 4.8

This maximum expiratory flow volume curve was obtained from a 10-year-old child with breathing difficulties.

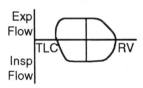

1. What does this maximum expiratory flow volume curve suggest?

Question 4.9

A preterm infant of 25 weeks gestation is being nursed in an incubator set to a temperature of 37°C, but at 48 h of age is found to be cold (rectal temperature 35.2°C). Plasma results are:

Sodium	162 mmol/l
Potassium	5.3 mmol/l
Urea	15.0 mmol/l
Glucose	7.2 mmol/l

1. What is the likely cause of the biochemical abnormalities?
2. What two measures would you institute to correct this?

Question 4.10

An infant presented with dehydration due to diarrhoea. This solution was available:

Sodium	90 mmol/l
Potassium	20 mmol/l
Chloride	80 mmol/l
Citrate	10 mmol/l
Glucose	2%

1. Is this solution safe to use in this child?

Paper 4.1 *ANSWERS*

Answer 4.1

1. Right optic tract
   Both optic radiations emanating from the lateral geniculate body
   Lateral geniculate body itself
2. Lesion in the right temporal lobe damaging the temporal lobe radiation

Discussion

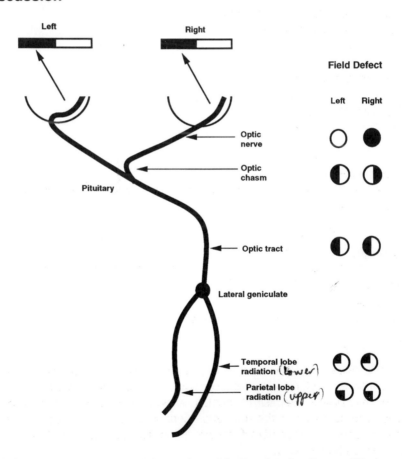

This figure shows the field defects alongside the visual pathway. Blindness in one eye represents retinal or optic nerve dysfunction, e.g. the optic nerve is involved in optic neuritis, producing unilateral blindness. It may also be involved by tumour or undergo atrophy secondary to prolonged raised intracranial pressure.

Bitemporal hemianopoia is classically found in patients with a craniopharyngioma or pituitary tumour secondary to pressure on the optic chiasm. The optic radiations fan out from the lateral geniculate bodies and travel in the temporal and parietal lobes before reaching their destination in the occipital lobe. Lesions in the temporal lobe may give a homonymous superior field defect if the optic radiations are affected. Similarly, a lesion in the parietal lobe may show an inferior homonymous field defect.   *quadrantopia*

The pupillary response is affected only if fibres proximal to the lateral geniculate body, in the midbrain, or third nerve are damaged.

Answer 4.2

1. Generalized ECG low voltage trace
2. Incorrect standardization
   Obesity or thick chest wall ✓
   Emphysema
   Pericardial effusion ✓
   Constrictive pericarditis
   Myxoedema
   Hypopituitarism

Further reading

Park M K, Guntheroff W G 1992 How to interpret pediatric ECGs, 2nd edn. Mosby Yearbook, St Louis

Answer 4.3

1. Patent ductus arteriosus
2. None
   Left ventricular and left atrial hypertrophy

Discussion

This child has a patent ductus arteriosus, which can be detected by cross-sectional and Doppler echocardiography, so catheterization is now seldom necessary. Persistent ductus arteriosus probably represents a structural abnormality in the ductus present at birth. It is the second most common congenital heart defect, accounting for approximately 10% of all such defects in full-term infants.

In the fetal circulation, the ductus allows right ventricular blood to bypass the non-expanded and non-ventilated lungs. Both the low PaO_2 of the blood and high levels of circulating prostaglandins in the fetus inhibit constriction of the ductus. Expansion of the lungs occurring immediately upon delivery in the newborn results in most of the right heart blood and, in turn, pulmonary artery blood being diverted immediately to the now 'lower in resistance' pulmonary

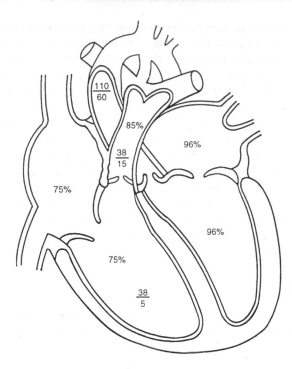

vascular bed. This flow through the lungs allows the circulating prostaglandins in the fetus to be cleared by the most effective system, the lungs, and immediately allows oxygenation of blood, thus increasing the circulating PaO$_2$. The decreased prostaglandins and increased blood PaO$_2$ result in the normal constriction of the ductus. The ductus is closed functionally by 72 h of age and sealed structurally by 3 months.

If the ductus remains open and the pulmonary resistance gradually drops after birth, blood flows from the aorta through the ductus and into the pulmonary arteries. With normal pulmonary resistance, flow through the ductus begins during mid to late systole and continues through diastole. The diameter of a clinically detectable ductus ranges from <1 mm to >1 cm at the narrowest diameter.

In an uncomplicated patent ductus there is a pure volume workload placed on the left heart with little or no effect on the right heart. The additional work on the left ventricle depends directly on the size of the persistent ductus and the result of flow through it. The additional blood volume from the ductus mixes with blood ejected from the right ventricle into the pulmonary artery. In the absence of increased pulmonary resistance, however, this extra blood does not add significantly to the work of the right ventricle. There are usually no physical or clinical laboratory signs suggesting right-sided involvement.

The ECG may be normal. With a larger ductus, left ventricular hypertrophy and left atrial enlargement may be seen. A chest X-ray may show cardiomegaly which is proportionate to the size of the ductus, and there may be plethora. The actual ductus can usually be visualized by echocardiography. At the same time, other intracardiac lesions associated with the ductus can be ruled out. The continuous wave Doppler can detect small streams of abnormal flow in the pulmonary artery, including the tiny flow from a ductus that is too small to be audible or visualized by echo; the tiny abnormal jet of blood can be visualized by a colour Doppler.

If there is any doubt with regards to the diagnosis, a cardiac catheter is usually performed. Catheterization of a patient with a patent ductus arteriosus will show an increase in oxygen saturation of blood in the main pulmonary artery. During catheterization the catheter may pass from the pulmonary artery through the ductus into the descending aorta. The presence of a ductus arteriosus should be confirmed by an angiocardiogram recorded on the lateral view with injection of contrast in the descending aorta immediately adjacent to the usual entrance site of the ductus. This provides details about the size and exact shape of the ductus.

Further reading

Campbell A G M, McIntosh N (eds) 1992 Forfar and Arneil's Textbook of paediatrics, 4th edn. Churchill Livingstone, Edinburgh, pp. 227–228

Answer 4.4

1. Down's syndrome (47 XX+21)
2. Low level
3. 1 in 700 (acceptable answers would range from 1 in 600 to 1 in 750)
4. 1 in 100

Discussion

Down's syndrome affects approximately 1 in 700 babies. There is a well recognized association with advancing maternal age, with the incidence rising to 1% when the mother is 40 years. Advanced paternal age has very little effect.

The most striking feature in the neonate is hypotonia and, although the diagnosis is usually evident at this time, it may sometimes be missed if the baby is very preterm. In infants and older children the most characteristic features are upward sloping palpebral fissures and protruding tongue, single palmar creases, mild short stature and mild-to-moderate developmental delay. IQ scores range from 25 to 70 and social skills often exceed other intellectual parameters.

Life expectancy in Down's syndrome has improved dramatically as a result of the widespread availablity of antibiotics. Approximately 15–20% of Down's children die before 5 years, usually as a result of severe inoperable congenital heart disease. Life expectancy for the remainder is well into adult life. By the age of 40 years almost all individuals with Down's will have developed Alzheimer's disease.

Further reading
Hull D, Johnson D I 1993 Essential paediatrics, 3rd edn. Churchill
Livingstone, Edinburgh, pp. 14–15

Answer 4.5

1. Bacterial meningitis due to *Listeria monocytogenes*
2. Ampicillin and gentamicin intravenously

Discussion

The CSF pattern of increased polymorphs, glucose <60% of plasma value and elevated protein are all consistent with septic meningitis. In an immunocompromized child, if Gram-positive bacilli are seen in the CSF, the pathogenic organism is likely to be *Listeria monocytogenes*. This bacillus may be mistaken for a contaminant as diptheroids are common on the skin but Gram-stain findings should never be dismissed as contaminants if there is CSF pleocytosis or abnormal biochemical findings. The red cells are due to a traumatic tap and a rough correction can be made for this by comparing the numbers of red and white cells in the CSF with those of peripheral blood. In this case, the ratio in peripheral blood is about 500 red cells for every white cell and therefore the presence of 20 red cells/µl in the CSF cannot explain the 720 white cells.

Neonates and the immunosuppressed are most vulnerable to listeria, via the transplacental or gastrointestinal routes. The latter can occur from contaminated food. A mononuclear reaction (hence 'monocytogenes') occurs in the blood of rabbits but, in contrast, increased numbers of polymorphonuclear leucocytes is a more usual finding in the peripheral blood of infected humans.

Non-Hodgkin's lymphoma accounts for 5% of all childhood cancers and may involve the B and T cells, in the latter case leading to depressed cell-mediated immunity, which predisposes to viral and fungal infections. *Pneumocystis carinii* or measles pneumonia should prompt a search for: Di George syndrome, Wiskott-Aldrich syndrome, ataxia telangectasia, chronic mucocutaneous candidiasis, severe combined immune deficiency and lymphoma, all of which are associated with impaired T-cell immunity.

Ampicillin *and* an aminoglycoside are the treatment of choice because they are synergistic against *Listeria monocytogenes*. A broad-spectrum cephalosporin such as cefotaxime would be reasonable empirical therapy while there is uncertainty about the infecting organisms, but the question specifically asks for the therapy of choice if diagnosis is confirmed. Equal marks would be awarded for 'aminoglycoside', 'gentamicin' or any other aminoglycoside provided this is combined with ampicillin and both are given intravenously. Examiners do not expect precise drug dosages to be given.

Answer 4.6

1. Recent blood transfusion
   Mixed deficiency of iron and folic acid or B_{12}
   Chronic haemolytic anaemia without folic acid supplementation
   Primary sideroblastic anaemia
2. Serum ferritin
   Serum B_{12}
   Red cell folate
   Reticulocyte count (or other test suggestive of haemolysis)

Discussion

The child has a mild degree of anaemia with a normal mean corpuscular volume but a dimorphic blood film. Red blood cells have a median survival of 120 days because all mature red cells lack a nucleus and are therefore destined for cell death. Once the cells become old they are cleared away by the reticuloendothelial system and in particular the spleen. At any one time in the circulation, therefore, there are cells of many different ages and the usual explanation of a dimorphic blood film is that two populations of red cells have arisen at different points in time but both within the last 120 days. Most blood counts are done by automated counters rather than by hand and therefore, although there may be a dimorphic blood film, the mean corpuscular volume may be calculated as normal.

If a child with a microcytic hypochromic iron-deficiency anaemia is transfused because the degree of anaemia is severe (either severely symptomatic, haemoglobin <4.0 g/dl, or non-compliance with iron therapy), the blood film will contain a mixture of the smaller iron-deficient red cells and the donor cells of normal size and haemoglobin content.

Both folic acid and B_{12} deficiency are very rare in children in the UK but if either of these occurs serially with iron deficiency (either through serial nutritional deficiences or because the gastrointestinal disease leading to malabsorption of folic acid or B_{12} is complicated by blood loss), there will be populations of both the hypochromic microcytic iron-deficient red cells and the macrocytic red cells of the megaloblastic anaemias.

If there is active haemolysis, iron deficiency does not occur as the iron obtained from the destroyed red cells can be recycled. However, aggressive haemolysis may unmask folic acid deficiency and for this reason neonates who have had an exchange transfusion for a haemolytic anaemia are discharged on folic acid 0.25 mg/kg/day until 6 weeks of age. Children with hereditary spherocytosis remain on folic acid until splenectomy is performed. As there is no evidence in the blood film of a pancytopenia, if the cause of the dimorphic film is a haemolytic process, this is not due to hypersplenism but is more likely to be due to an isolated red cell anomaly. As the blood film did not report abnormal numbers of spherocytes or eliptocytes, the most likely cause would be a haemoglobinopathy or enzymopathy rather than a membranopathy. Whatever the appearances of the original population of red cells, a prolonged period of haemolysis may lead to folic acid deficiency and the appearance of a population of macrocytes.

All causes of megaloblastic anaemia in children are rare but folic acid deficiency is much commoner than B_{12} deficiency in childhood. Because of the relative amounts of each substance stored in the body, it would take over a year of complete absence of absorption of B_{12} before any ill-effects were noted; iron stores last a few months, but folic acid stores are in constant need of replenishment and megaloblastic anaemia may develop within 6–8 weeks of the onset of folic acid deficiency. Breast milk contains enough folic acid for the normally developing child but if preterm infants are not supplemented with oral folate they are a particularly vulnerable group. Folic acid is absorbed in the upper jejunum and therefore small bowel malabsorption, including coeliac disease, may lead to deficiency. Trimethoprim is a folic acid antagonist and should not be given to infants <42 weeks post-conceptional age because of the risk of inducing an effective folic acid deficiency. Long-term anticonvulsant therapy (phenytoin and barbiturates) is also associated with folic acid deficiency. In gluten-sensitive enteropathy, anaemia is most often due to iron deficiency but megaloblastic anaemia due to folate deficiency may also occur.

A dimorphic blood film can occur in sideroblastic anaemia, which is characterized by an inability to utilize iron, although iron is present in sufficient amounts. The typical features, therefore, are of anaemia in the peripheral blood film, but iron overload in other tissues. Bone marrow biopsy will show the presence of so-called 'ring sideroblasts'. In the congenital form, the film is usually hypochromic and microcytic and this is an X-linked disorder. An acquired sideroblastic anaemia may either be idiopathic or secondary to drugs, in particular isoniazid used to treat tuberculosis. In the acquired form the dimorphic blood film is a mixture of normocytic cells and microcytic cells.

The four investigations that would distinguish the above are:

a) serum ferritin which will be low in iron-deficiency anaemia and very high in an iron-loading disorder such as sideroblastic anaemia;
b) serum B_{12} will be low in B_{12} deficiency;
c) red cell folate will be low in folate deficiency;
d) a reticulocyte count which will be high if there is an active haemolytic process.

Further reading

Campbell A G M, McIntosh N (eds) 1992 Forfar and Arneil's Textbook of paediatrics, 4th edn. Churchill Livingstone, Edinburgh, pp. 922–925, 937

Answer 4.7

1. Microangiopathic haemolytic anaemia

2. Plamsa bilirubin
   Direct Coombs' test
   Reticulocyte count
   Urinary urobilinogen
   Plasma haptoglobulins
3. Haemolytic uraemic syndrome

Discussion

The low haemoglobin and platelet count are suggestive of a microangiopathic haemolytic anaemia. The presence of schistocytes — abnormal distorted fragmented red cells — is a result of red cell shredding through fibrin strands deposited in small blood vessels. This can occur in disseminated intravascular coagulation but the normal clotting studies preclude this diagnosis. The consumption of platelets occurs because of the formation of microthrombi within the circulation.

The diagnosis will be supported by:

a) elevated unconjugated bilirubin in the plasma, confirming haemolysis of red cells;
b) a negative direct Coombs' test, confirming that the cause of the haemolysis is mechanical rather than immunological;
c) an increased reticulocyte count which will demonstrate that the low haemoglobin and platelet count were not due to marrow failure;
d) a raised urobilinogen in the urine;
e) a reduction in free plasma haptoglobulins, the carrier protein for haemoglobin and haemoglobinuria, which indicates intravascular haemolysis.

The raised plasma urea suggests that the cause is haemolytic uraemic syndrome, which is the classic childhood example of microangiopathic haemolytic anaemia. A similar picture may occur with grafts or prosthetic heart valves when there is a purely mechanical disruption of the red cells within the larger vessels.

The most likely bleeding sites in this condition are epistaxis, bleeding from the gums, haematuria and purpura (all associated with low platelet counts), as opposed to bleeding into the joints, muscles and subcutaneous bruising, which are features of a coagulopathy (e.g. haemophilia).

Haemolytic uraemic syndrome may occur sporadically (in which case the child is usually older and has a worse prognosis) or in epidemics, often in association with verotoxins produced by a particular strain of *Escherichia coli*. Early aggressive management is thought to improve the prognosis with respect to neurological outcome. Therefore, the child should be transferred to a centre where dialysis can be undertaken for acute renal failure and at this time the anaemia will be corrected.

The prognosis depends on the duration of the anuria. Up to 10% may die, most of the others will recover fully, but 1–3% will progress to chronic renal failure. In some series, up to 10% of survivors have chronic neurological sequelae.

Further reading
Campbell A G M, McIntosh N (eds) 1992 Forfar and Arneil's Textbook of paediatrics, 4th edn. Churchill Livingstone, Edinburgh, pp. 927–928, 935

Answer 4.8

1. Fixed airways obstruction

Discussion

Maximum expiratory flow volume curves are the pulmonary function tests of choice in diagnosing upper airways obstruction. They can define the site of obstruction as well as documenting its presence. Because the shape of the flow-volume curve carries significant information, and often in a subtle manner, it is important to examine the curve and avoid strict reliance on numbers extracted from it.

With a fixed obstruction, plateau and limitation of flow is seen both during inspiration and expiration, as in this case. Patients with obstructing lesions of the upper airway can go unrecognized and misdiagnosed if pulmonary function testing is not examined closely. They may sometimes be confused with asthma as they are often seen with wheezing, shortness of breath or even hypoxia. Fixed lesions do not allow the airways to change cross-sectional area regardless of the change in transmural pressure. In normal individuals, the maximum airflow achieved during the first 25% of a force vital capacity manoeuvre is directly dependent on effort. With upper airway obstruction, flow at high lung volumes becomes limited much earlier by the obstruction and produces changes early in forced expiration.

With variable lesions, however, the size of the airway does respond to changes in transmural pressure. Variable extra-thoracic obstruction produces flow limitation and a plateau only on inspiration. With this type of lesion, intramural pressure during expiration is much higher than pressure outside the lumen (atmospheric pressure). This actually causes the airway to dilate in the area of obstruction during the expiratory manoeuvre. The obstruction is thus only obvious on the inspiratory portion of the flow volume curve (A). This is why stridor (e.g. croup or epiglottitis) is predominantly an inspiratory sound.

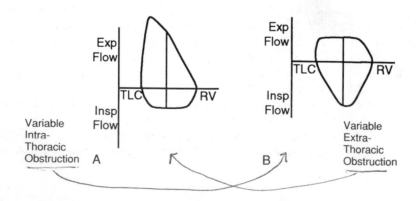

Variable intrathoracic obstruction causes flow limitation and a plateau only on expiration, because the pressure outside the lumen (plural pressure) becomes much greater than intraluminal pressure (B). Hence, expiratory wheeze is typical of asthma and bronchiolitis.

It should be noted that patients with bilateral obstruction of both main bronchii can have pulmonary function changes identical to patients with intrathoracic upper airways obstruction.

Answer 4.9

1. Excessive transepidermal water loss
2. Correct hypovolaemia with 10 ml/kg 4% human albumin solution
   Increase daily free water intake

Discussion

At 48 h of age, the skin of such a preterm infant remains extremely thin and the dead layer, the stratum corneum, which acts as a barrier to prevent water loss, is still poorly formed. Transepidermal water loss is therefore high and can reach 120 ml/kg/day, depending on gestational age, postnatal age and the ambient humidity. Below 36 weeks gestation, sweating does not appear until a few days after birth and even then remains limited compared with a term infant or an older child. Before 30 weeks gestation, sweating is absent in the first 2 weeks of life and can be ignored in fluid balance considerations. Because of the combination of increased transepidermal water loss and no sweating, the insensible fluid that is lost is free water rather than isotonic. The result is a total body free water deficit and plasma hypernatraemia and hyperosmolality. In addition, the total body free water deficit is associated with a contraction in the intravascular volume, which will lead to hypotension, acidosis, decreased renal blood flow and glomerular filtration rate, explaining the high urea. Creatinine concentration in the plasma of infants in the first 48 h of life is more difficult to interpret as it mirrors the much higher maternal plasma creatinine immediately prior to delivery. The relatively high plasma glucose concentration probably reflects a stress reaction to the hypovolaemia which will trigger a release of cortisol and catecholamines, both insulin antagonists.

With this degree of hypernatraemia, this infant is at risk of seizures and in addition the high urea suggests that organ perfusion will be poor. However, over rapid correction of either the hypernatraemia or the hypovolaemia may be dangerous. Plasma volumes should be expanded initially with 10 ml/kg of 4% human albumin solution and this may need to be repeated. The plasma sodium should be brought down gradually over the next 48 h by increasing the amount of free water given each day. Many preterm infants are started on a regimen which gradually increases from 60 ml/kg/day over the first 24 h up to 150 ml/kg/day by 4 days. However, in very preterm infants, this incremental regimen may need to be accelerated and, especially for infants nursed under radiant warmers, fluid requirements of 300–400 ml/kg/day may be required in the first few days. A third measure, which would not improve the situation acutely but which might have prevented it from arising, is to place the infant inside a humidified body box as this reduces the transepidermal water loss.

An important point is that at all ages throughout childhood, hypernatraemia is much more commonly due to water depletion than sodium overload. In the neonatal period, sodium overload is usually iatrogenic as a result of the administration of hypertonic solutions but in the older child may be a feature of Munchausen by Proxy syndrome due to parental administration of saline orally.

Further reading

Campbell A G M, McIntosh N (eds) 1992 Forfar and Arneil's Textbook of paediatrics, 4th edn. Churchill Livingstone, Edinburgh, pp. 158–165
Costarina A, Baumgart S 1986 Modern fluid and electrolyte management of critically ill premature infants. Pediatric Clinics of North America 33: 153–178

Answer 4.10

1. Yes

Discussion

Oral rehydration will succed in almost all children who are not shocked if appropriate fluids are given in an appropriate way. Physiological studies in cholera have led to the formulation of oral rehydration fluids which have also been shown to be suitable for all infectious cases of diarrhoea. The solution described is the WHO recommended solution for oral rehydration. The most important items are the sodium and glucose concentrations (see table, in mmol/l). A nasogastric tube may be used to achieve a steady infusion of fluid if vomiting or food refusal is a major problem.

	Sodium	Chloride	Potassium	Bicarbonate	Glucose
WHO-UNICEF	90	80	20	30	110
Dextrolyte	35	30	13	18*	200
Dioralyte	60	60	20	10+	90
Rehydrat	50	50	20	20	91#

* As lactate; # Also contains 8 mmol/l citric acid and 94 mmol/l sucrose; + As citrate

Paper 5 *QUESTIONS*

Question 5.1

This is the ECG rhythm strip from a newborn baby.

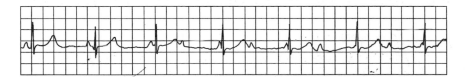

1. What abnormality does it show?
2. Give two possible causes for such an ECG trace.

Question 5.2

A child with suspected developmental delay could build this tower of 1" blocks and unbutton front buttons.

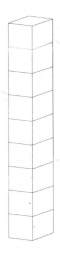

1. At what age would you expect a normal child to accomplish these tasks?

Question 5.3

These are the results of a cardiac catheter performed on a 12-year-old girl with heart disease.

	Oxygen saturation (%)	Blood pressure (mmHg) (systolic/diastolic)
Right atrium	60	
Right ventricle	65	100/10
Pulmonary artery	70	100/60
Left atrium	96	
Left ventricle	80	100/10
Aorta	80	100/70

1. What is the diagnosis?
2. The child's haematocrit was 75%. What treatment may be required?

Question 5.4

The karyotype is reported as 46 XX, −15, +t (15q21q). The parents want to know the result of this investigation.

1. What will you tell them?

Question 5.5

A 12-year-old British child spent 4 months in northern Nigeria. He was well until 2 weeks after return to the UK, when he developed rigors. Ring forms of *Plasmodium falciparum* were seen in the blood film. After he was given a standard course of chloroquine, his symptoms resolved completely. He was well until 6 weeks later, when he again developed rigors. Throat swab, blood culture and urine culture were negative. Chest radiograph was normal.

1. What is the most likely cause of his fever?
2. How should this be treated?

Question 5.6

These results were obtained from a 9-month-old infant with recurrent bruising and purpura.

Haemoglobin	10.5 g/dl
Platelet count	$45 \times 10^9/l$

Blood film	Normal red and white cells, large platelets
Bleeding time	17 min (normal <7 min)
Platelet aggregation	Normal with adrenaline and arachidonic acid, defective with ristocetin

1. What is the likely diagnosis?

Question 5.7

A woman, known to be pregnant with twins, begins labour spontaneously at 29 weeks gestation. The first twin is a boy who requires oxygen for the first hour of life only. His packed cell volume at 1 h is 65%. Cord prolapse follows delivery of the first twin and the second is born by emergency caesarian section, being delivered 16 min after the cord prolapse. This girl has an Apgar score of 3 following delivery and requires positive pressure ventilation from birth. At 1 h the haemoglobin concentration is 12 g/dl.

1. What is the most likely cause of the ventilation requirement in the second twin?
2. Give the most likely reason why the haemoglobin is 12 g/dl in the second twin.

Question 5.8

A 10-year-old boy was admitted to hospital with a clinical diagnosis of right lower lobe pneumonia. Two days before, he produced purulent sputum that was tinged with bright red blood. The child developed right pleuritic chest pain. Microscopy of the sputum showed only pus cells, and culture was negative. Blood culture was negative. There was no history of foreign travel, or close contact with birds. The following results were obtained:

Haemoglobin	12.8 g/dl
White cell count	$9.7 \times 10^9/l$
Neutrophils	89%
Blood film	Normal
Plasma:	
Urea	11.0 mmol/l
Creatinine	Normal
Electrolytes	Normal
Arterial blood gases:	
pH	7.42
PaO_2	8.2 kPa
$PaCO_2$	4.2 kPa

A chest radiograph showed consolidation of the right lower lobe with substantial loss of volume and a small pleural effusion.

1. Suggest three likely diagnoses.
2. Give two investigations.

Question 5.9

A neonatal patient suddenly developed cyanosis. There were no obvious respiratory or cardiac causes to account for the cyanosis. The following results were obtained:

Haemoglobin	14 g/dl
White cell count	10×10^9/l
Platelet count	300×10^9/l

The patient's blood was brown in colour and did not become red on exposure to air.

1. What is the likely diagnosis?
2. What three other measurements would help confirm your suspicions?

Question 5.10

An 8-year-old child was admitted with the following investigations:

Plasma sodium	128 mmol/l
Plasma potassium	4.0 mmol/l
Plasma creatinine	50 µmol/l
Plasma urea	12 mmol/l
Haemoglobin	14.0 g/dl
White cell count	8×10^9/l
Platelet count	250×10^9/l

He had had diarrhoea and was transferred to you because a diagnosis of renal failure due to haemolytic uraemic syndrome is suspected. The last urine passed 12 h ago contained a urinary sodium of 5 mmol/l and urinary urea of 80 mmol/l.

1. What would be your immediate fluid management of this child?

Paper 5 ANSWERS

Answer 5.1

1. Complete heart block (third degree)
2. Isolated finding
   Associated with structural abnormalities, e.g. transposition of the great vessels
   Maternal systemic lupus erythematosus
   Post infarction
   Post cardiac surgery

Discussion

In complete atrioventricular block, the atria and ventricles beat independently of each other. The ventricular rate is usually regular but slow. The ventricular complex is normal if the pacemaker is in the atrioventricular node or at a level higher than the bifurcation of the bundle of His. Most children with congenital complete heart block have normal ventricular complexes. In surgically induced or acquired (post infarction) third degree heart block, the QRS complexes have the appearance of ventricular premature beats, i.e. the complex is wide and of abnormal morphology.

In this case, the mother had systemic lupus erythematosus. Complete heart block in the newborn is the only arrhythmia associated with immunological disease. Transfer of anti-Ro across the placenta variably results in congenital heart block. Most mothers have no symptoms of systemic lupus erythematosus at this time. In those infants who die, IgG and complement deposits in cardiac conducting tissue and muscle can be found. Infants may also develop neonatal lupus skin lesions. Subsequent infants may be affected if maternal anti-Ro persists. Anti-nuclear antibody is a less sensitive test than anti-Ro, since Ro antibody characterizes a particular form of anti-nuclear-antibody-negative systemic lupus erythematosus.

Further reading
   Watson J G, Bird A J 1989 Handbook of immunological investigations in children. Wright, Bristol

Answer 5.2

1. 3 years old

Discussion

A 3-year-old child should be able to:

— go upstairs one foot per step, and downstairs with two feet per step ;
— jump off the bottom step;
— stand on one foot for a few seconds;
— ride a tricycle;
— be trusted to carry 'inexpensive' china and so help set the table.

Answer 5.3

1. Eisenmenger's syndrome
2. Venesection

Discussion

Pulmonary hypertension has developed causing bidirectional shunting. The child has a large ventricular septal defect and has developed Eisenmenger's syndrome. Cardiac lesions likely to lead to Eisenmenger's syndrome are those that allow high pulmonary blood flow in the presence of high pulmonary pressures, such as large defects of the ventricular septum and atrioventricular canal defects. Presence of hypoxia, such as that occurring with truncus arteriosus, hastens the development of pulmonary vascular disease. Defects with low pulmonary pressures, such as atrial septal defects, are much less likely to lead to Eisenmenger's syndrome and, despite their high rate of pulmonary blood flow, are usually tolerated for decades.

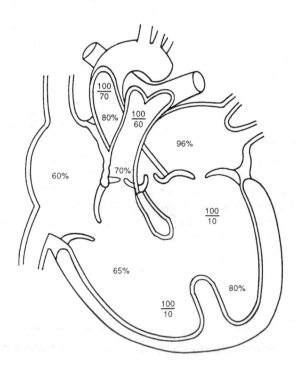

As obstructive pulmonary vascular disease develops, resistance increases in the pulmonary vascular bed. Venous blood follows the course of least resistance and is shunted away from the pulmonary arteries through the cardiac defect into the systemic circulation. This results in hypoxia. The greater the pulmonary resistance or the lower the systemic resistance, the greater will be the right-to-left shunting of blood.

At the time of diagnosis of heart disease, the clinical presentation is usually that of congestive heart failure due to a high pulmonary blood flow. As the pulmonary vascular resistance increases, the signs and symptoms of congestive cardiac failure decrease. When pulmonary resistance exceeds systemic resistance, hypoxia occurs and progresses as the pulmonary vascular resistance continues to rise.

The following signs are typical of patients with pulmonary hypertension. The precordium is hyperdynamic and the second heart sound is very loud and frequently palpable at the upper left sternal border. This is due to the pulmonary component of the second sound. Splitting of the second sound is generally absent. Murmurs are usually soft because the intracardiac defects are large with little pressure gradient between the chambers. Cyanosis and clubbing of the fingers may be present.

In early mild cases, cardiac catheterization is often required to make the diagnosis of obstructive pulmonary vascular disease. This is important as there are few cardiac lesions that cannot be corrected or palliated surgically in the absence of advanced pulmonary vascular disease.

Polycythemia is usually found after the onset of a significant right-to-left shunt, and will increase as hypoxia worsens. Interestingly, because of the increased iron demands, red cell indices frequently show indications of relative iron-deficiency anaemia despite an overall polycythemia. Blood viscosity has been shown to increase exponentially with haematocrit. The crucial range appears to be an haematocrit of 70–75%, at which level blood viscosity increases dramatically. Studies have suggested that both systemic and especially pulmonary vascular resistance increase exponentially with haematocrit as a result of the increase in viscosity. Coronary artery blood flow also decreases significantly as haematocrit increases.

The haemoglobin status of patients is monitored regularly. An increased blood haemoglobin content is required to maintain systemic oxygen delivery in a normal range as hypoxemia increases. This is beneficial as long as the haematocrit does not rise above 60–65%. Above this level, because of the problems with blood viscosity described, venesection is performed to lower the haematocrit. Anaemia should also be avoided in these patients as it compromises oxygen delivery.

Answer 5.4

1. Down's syndrome due to an unbalanced Robertsonian translocation

Discussion

The karyotype shows that the patient is female (46 XX) with Down's syndrome, due to the replacement of a normal number 15 chromosome (indicated by the −15) with a translocation chromosome consisting of the fused long arms of a number 15 chromosome (15q) and the number 21 chromosome (21q). Another example of this kind of notation is the use of 5p minus to refer to the Cri-du-Chat syndrome. This means that there is loss of or deletion of a small portion of chromosomal genetic material from the end of the short arm of a number 5 chromosome.

When a child has Down's syndrome as a result of an unbalanced Robertsonian translocation there is a 25% probability that one of the parents will carry this in a balanced form. The parent is therefore, phenotypically normal. The other 75% of cases arise as de novo events and have a low recurrence risk of approximately 1%. If, however, a parent is a balanced carrier, there is a significant risk of a future child being affected, usually 2–5% for a carrier male and 10–15% for a carrier female. It is therefore important that parental chromosome studies are undertaken to elucidate the risk. However, the implications of this should be explained to the parents and some parents decline as they may not wish to know which of them was responsible for the abnormality in their offspring.

In the very rare event that a parent carries a balanced 21q21q Robertsonian translocation, the risk of Down's syndrome in liveborn offspring will, of course, be 100% as there is no normal 21 chromosome to inherit.

Unbalanced Robertsonian translocations account for only 3% of all Down's syndrome. Another 2% are due to mosaicism and the phenotypic severity depends on the proportion of cells which are trisomic. If this Down's syndrome individual should go on to have children, there is a relatively high risk that the baby will have full Trisomy 21 with the precise risk equalling the proportion of gametes which carry the additional 21 chromosome. The other 95% of Down's syndrome are due to Trisomy 21 due to non-dysjunction and the additional number 21 chromosome derived from the mother in 80% of cases. If a woman with Down's syndrome due to Trisomy 21 conceives, there is a 50% risk that the baby will also have Trisomy 21. Males with Down's syndrome have rarely, if ever, reproduced.

Further reading

Campbell A G M, McIntosh N (eds) 1992 Forfar and Arneil's Textbook of paediatrics, 4th edn. Churchill Livingstone, Edinburgh, pp. 60–63

Answer 5.5

1. *Plasmodium vivax* malaria

Malaria

2. Choloroquine and primaquine

Chloroquine
Primaquine

Discussion

In this context, the most likely cause of an intermittent fever is malaria. *Plasmodium falciparum* malaria was diagnosed initially, and was treated successfully with chloroquine, therefore drug resistance is most unlikely. Recurrence is likely to be with non-falciparum malaria, as this will not have been eradicated by chloroquine in the exo-erythrocytic stage. *P. vivax* is the most likely candidate. In vivax malaria, usually the spleen and, particularly in children, the liver becomes enlarged and tender. Treatment should be with a further course of chloroquine followed by primaquine. Malaria prophylaxis should always be continued for 4–6 weeks after return from an endemic region.

Malaria is a protozoal disease (as are amoebiasis, giardiasis, Leishmaniasis, trypanosomiasis and toxoplasmosis) which requires human hosts, mosquito carriers and suitable temperature and humidity to become endemic. The interval between being bitten by an infected mosquito and the onset of fever is about 1 week for falciparum malaria and longer for other types. Occasionally the first attack occurs months later, particularly if an incomplete course of suppressive drugs has been taken. Falciparum infections are potentially the most severe and cerebral malaria, blackwater fever (due to intravascular haemolysis) and acute renal failure are dangerous complications. Children may die suddenly.

The commonest tropical disease to be imported to the UK in children is malaria, then typhoid. Malaria can only be spread by a vector, the anopheline mosquito, or by transfusion or inoculation of infected blood. Generally, therefore, the child must have travelled abroad to contract the disease. In contrast, diseases such as typhoid, dysentry and tuberculosis can be passed by an infected relative visiting or returning from abroad. Hence, such diseases are more commonly seen in children from Asian families.

Answer 5.6

1. Bernard–Soulier syndrome

Discussion

Bernard–Soulier syndrome is an autosomal recessive disease with giant platelets on the blood film and usually a moderate bleeding tendency. Inherited deficiency of platelet membrane glycoprotein 1B leads to absent aggregation with ristocetin, which does not correct with normal plasma. The deficiency results in the inability to bind Von Willebrand's factor or ristocetin. As in Glanzmann's thrombasthenia, platelet transfusion is the only means of therapy. However, problems with platelet infusions may occur, due to the development of antibodies against the glycoprotein 1B in the transfused platelets.

Further reading
Campbell A G M, McIntosh N (eds) 1992 Forfar and Arneil's Textbook of paediatrics, 4th edn. Churchill Livingstone, Edinburgh, pp. 948–950

Answer 5.7

1. Birth asphyxia exacerbating hyaline membrane disease

Hyaline membrane disease
Respiratory distress syndrome
Surfactant deficiency

2. Twin-to-twin transfusion syndrome

Discussion

At 29 weeks gestation, most infants will show signs of respiratory distress due to surfactant deficiency. Surfactant, is a surface tension lowering agent which increases lung compliance and prevents smaller alveoli coalescing into larger neighbouring alveoli. Surfactant deficiency is associated with stiff lungs, increased work of breathing, the failure to establish functional residual capacity, hypoxia due to ventilation perfusion mismatch, decreased alveolar surface area and increased thickness of the alveolar capillary membrane. The intrapartum asphyxia often associated with cord prolapse causes hypoxia and acidosis, which inhibit the enzymes responsible for surfactant synthesis.

The fact the twins are different sexes and therefore not identical does not exclude a twin-to-twin transfusion since they may still have vascular connections at placental level. A feto-maternal transfusion from the second twin would not explain the high packed cell volume in the first twin. At 1 h of age the infant is too young for periventricular haemorrhage to be likely unless due to a very traumatic delivery, in which case subdural haemorrhage is more likely. Disseminated intravascular coagulation secondary to birth asphyxia would be unlikely to drop the haemoglobin so quickly.

Answer 5.8

1. Pneumococcal pneumonia

Inhaled foreign body
Congenital lesion, e.g. pulmonary sequestration or bronchogenic cyst *with* secondary infection
Pulmonary tuberculosis
Lung malignancy

2. Microscopy and culture of pleural fluid
Thoracic CT scan
Bronchoscopy
Mantoux test

Discussion

Streptococcus pneumoniae is the commonest cause of lobar pneumonia in children in the UK. The raised plasma urea suggests dehydration, which is more consistent with an acutely ill child with a fever (although the temperature is not given) than the other diagnoses. Blood cultures are positive in approximately half the cases.

Tuberculosis is an unlikely diagnosis, although the lower lobe may be affected. Features of tuberculosis include cough, haemoptysis and fever, but the illness tends to be more prolonged.

Inhaled foreign body should always be considered whenever there is evidence of bronchial obstruction, and although typically seen in children aged 1–3 years, may occur at any time of life. Older children will usually give a history suggestive of aspiration but such an event may be forgotten.

Infection with mycoplasma is not uncommon as a cause of bilateral, patchy pneumonia in children of school age. However, in the case described, the clinical course, volume loss and haemoptysis render this diagnosis less likely.

Volume loss and haemoptysis suggest an obstructing and ulcerating lesion. Pulmonary metastases are rare in this age group but the possibility of testicular germ cell tumour should be considered. Primary pulmonary neoplasms (particularly carcinoid) are again rare in children but may occur, and present with cough, haemoptysis and pneumonia.

Examination of the pleural fluid may confirm a bacterial aetiology. If a foreign body is strongly suspected, bronchoscopy is the investigation of choice. Chest X-ray in expiration and inspiration or fluoroscopy are not as good but acceptable answers. If a neoplasm seems likely, CT should accurately delineate the site of obstruction, but bronchoscopy (either flexible or rigid) is required for histological or microbiological diagnosis. A ventilation-perfusion scan would simply show a matched defect at the base of the right lung in all these lesions and would be unhelpful.

Answer 5.9

1. Methaemoglobinaemia
2. Methaemoglobin measured by spectrophotometry
   Assay of methaemoglobin reductase
   Detection of abnormal methaemoglobin

Discussion

Methaemoglobinaemia syndrome should be considered when cyanosis occurs without respiratory or cardiac disease, where the arterial PaO_2 is normal and blood remains dark when mixed with air. Methaemoglobin is an oxidized form of haemoglobin. When the iron is in its ferric state (methaemoglobin), there is no complex with oxygen. Normally, <4% of a neonate's haemoglobin is methaemoglobin. Cyanosis is apparent at methaemoglobin levels of 10% of the total haemoglobin. Symptoms due to decreased oxygen transport are generally not apparent until 30–40% of haemoglobin is oxidized to methaemoglobin.

Patients may have an acquired or congenital methaemoglobinaemia. Congential methaemoglobinaemia may be due to haemoglobin M disorders or NADH-methaemoglobin reductase deficiency. In neonates only α-chain abnormalities causing haemoglobin M present. Heterozygotes for HbM have increased methaemoglobin levels and may be cyanosed. The homozygous state is incompatible with life. Heterozygotes with NADH-methaemoglobin reductase deficiency may develop methaemoglobinaemia when challenged with toxic agents. Homozygotes are usually cyanosed.

This patient had an acquired methaemoglobinaemia due to exposure to prilocaine. During the first weeks of life normal neonates are particularly susceptible to certain chemicals that oxidize iron haemoglobin because fetal haemoglobin is more readily oxidized to the ferric state than haemoglobin A and neonates have a transient deficiency in NADH-methaemoglobin reductase activity.

Another enzyme, NADPH-methaemoglobin reductase, by itself is unable significantly to reduce methaemoglobin. In the presence of methylene blue, however, this enzyme rapidly reduces methaemoglobin to the ferrous form. Neonatal drug-induced or NADH-methaemogloibin reductase deficiency varieties respond to methylene blue. Oral ascorbic acid may reduce methaemoglobin directly and is usually given.

Further reading

Roberton NRC (ed) 1992 Textbook of neonatology, 2nd edn. Churchill Livingstone, Edinburgh, p. 698

Answer 5.10

1. Immediate expansion of circulating volume with 20 ml/kg plasma or 0.9% saline over 30 min

Discussion

This child has pre-renal renal failure due to hypovolaemia and the correct fluid management is immediate administration of 20 ml/kg plasma or normal saline over the next 30 min. This may have to be repeated until clinical assessment or central venous pressure measurement suggests the child is normovolaemic and at this stage 2 mg/kg intravenous frusemide may also be given. Diuretics should never be given in pre-renal renal failure until the hypovolaemia has been corrected.

In the steady-state:

Urinary excretion of creatinine (glomerular filtration rate × plasma creatinine concentration) = endogenous creatinine production by the skeletal muscle

If glomerular filtration rate falls, plasma creatinine rises until a new steady-state is reached, when again creatinine production = creatinine excretion. Since creatinine production depends on muscle mass and not glomerular filtration rate, the plasma creatinine is inversely proportional to the glomerular filtration rate. If the glomerular filtration rate falls by 50%, plasma creatinine will eventually reach a new steady-state at twice the previous concentration. The normal range of creatinine is wide (for children 20–80 µmol/l), and thus a large fall in glomerular filtration rate may be accompanied by an increase in plasma creatinine such that this remains within the upper limit of the normal range.

Whilst urea secretion also varies with glomerular filtration rate, the relationship is not as simple as for creatinine. First, almost half the urea filtered in the Bowman's capsule is reabsorbed by the tubules and, in addition, urea reabsorption is increased in the presence of hypovolaemia. Consequently, although urea will rise as well as plasma creatinine, if the glomerular filtration rate is reduced, urea clearance is not an accurate estimation of glomerular filtration rate. Moreover, whereas creatinine production varies little on a daily basis as long as muscle mass remains fairly constant, urea production is not constant, decreasing with liver disease and increasing following a high protein intake, gastrointestinal bleeding or a hypercatabolic state (e.g. following severe burns or trauma). If urea reabsorption is increased because of volume depletion, there is an elevation in the plasma urea over and above that which is due to the reduced glomerular filtration rate.

In this case, the wrong diagnosis has been made. Although a diarrhoeal illness is often a precursor of haemolytic uraemic syndrome, the normal full blood count does not support this diagnosis and it is much more likely that isotonic fluid lost as diarrhoea has been replaed with ingested free water, leading to hyponatraemia. Volume replacement has been inadequate and, as a result of the homeostatic defence mechanisms to maintain blood pressure, splanchnic blood flow is reduced. As a result, renal blood flow is decreased and glomerular filtration rate is reduced; as the child's plasma creatinine in health is not given, the rise in creatinine cannot be deduced. In contrast, it can be seen that the urea concentration is almost double the upper limit of normal and is elevated out of proportion to the plasma creatinine. This combination of findings — a low urinary sodium concentration, a high urine:plasma urea ratio (>5), a low urine output and a urinary urea elevated out of proportion to plasma concentration — constitute the response of a normal kidney to effective circulating volume depletion. In contrast, a patient with established acute renal failure has a urinary sodium of >40 mmol/l and poorly concentrated urine with a urine:plasma urea ratio <4, and urinalysis will usually reveal some haematuria, proteinuria or casts. Hypovolaemia may also complicate established renal failure but in this case the kidney is unable to respond normally to the decreased effective circulating volume and despite the hypovolaemia the urine tends to have a high sodium concentration, similar osmolality to plasma, and the plasma urea and creatinine are increased.

Decreased circulating volume; urine sodium <10 mmol/l	Decreased circulating volume; urine sodium >20 mmol/l	Normal or increased circulating volume; urine sodium >20 mmol/l
Gastrointestinal losses	Diuretic excess	SIADH
Severe burns	Adrenal insufficiency	Psychogenic polydipsia
Oedema forming states	Salt wasting renal disease	Established renal failure
	Diuretic phase of acute renal failure	
	Postobstructive uropathy diuresis	
	Osmotic diuretics	

Further reading

Milner A D, Hull D 1992 Hospital paediatrics, 2nd edn. Churchill Livingstone, Edinburgh, pp. 32, 208–209

Paper 6 *QUESTIONS*

Question 6.1

This is the EEG from a 7-month-old child who had just fallen asleep. The child was being investigated for abnormal movements of his legs and arms.

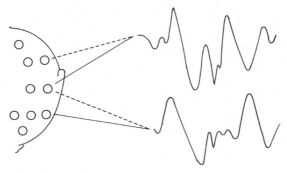

1. What does the EEG show?
2. What is the likely diagnosis?

Question 6.2

A 15-year-old boy presented to casualty with a small wound that had been contaminated with stable manure. His last reinforcing dose of tetanus immunization was 11 years ago.

1. What specific anti-tetanus treatment, if any, would you prescribe?

Question 6.3

This is the ECG trace from a 2-month-old infant who had become unwell recently and was found on examination to have a large liver, and on chest X-ray cardiomegaly.

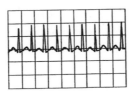

1. What does the ECG show?
2. Give two ways of treating this child's immediate problem.

Question 6.4

These are the results from a cardiac catheter performed on a 7-year-old child.

	Oxygen saturation (%)	Blood pressure (mmHg) (systolic/diastolic)
Right atrium	75	—/3
Right ventricle	75	25/3
Pulmonary artery	75	25/10
Left atrium	96	—/7
Left ventricle	96	100/7
Aorta	96	100/70

1. The child's parents are keen to know the result. What will you tell them?

Question 6.5

A 5-year-old boy attending his GP because of an upper respiratory tract infection was noted to be pale. Investigation revealed the following results:

Haemoglobin	9 g/dl
Mean corpuscular volume	61 fl
Mean corpuscular haemoglobin	19 pg
Mean corpuscular haemoglobin concentration	25 g/dl
Platelet count	$420 \times 10^9/l$
Serum ferritin	8 μg/l (normal 18–82 μg/l)
Transferrin saturation	Decreased

1. What do the investigations reveal?
2. What is the diagnosis?
3. What blood film changes are typically seen in such patients?

Question 6.6

A 3-kg boy was delivered by caesarian section. He was noted to be pale following delivery and a transplacental haemorrhage was suspected. The following blood results were obtained:

Haemoglobin	7 g/dl
Direct Coombs' test	Negative
Blood film	Normal apart from occasional spherocytes

Blood group:

Mother	O Rh(D) positive
Baby	O Rh(D) positive
Kleihauer test	Positive

1. Are these results consitent with a transplacental haemorrhage?
2. What does a positive Kleihauer test detect?

Question 6.7

A 4-year-old child, well until 6 months of age, is failing to thrive. Musculoskeletal and neurological examination are entirely normal. Arterial blood gas results are:

	Awake	Asleep
$PaCO_2$	5.1 kPa	8.0 kPa
Base excess	+5.3 mmol/l	+5.4 mmol/l

1. What is the most likely diagnosis?
2. What two further investigations would be most helpful in further management?

Question 6.8

A 3-month-old infant is brought to your clinic because of poor weight gain. She weighs 4 kg and takes five bottle feeds of cows' milk formula in each 24 h period, averaging 4 fl oz each time. The girl has an older brother with eczema and on examination her only abnormality, apart from low weight, is infantile eczema. Blood tests show the following results:

Haemoglobin	9.4 g/dl
Platelet count	$314 \times 10^9/l$
White cell count	$8.1 \times 10^9/l$
Neutrophils	$4.58 \times 10^9/l$ (normal $2.0-7.5 \times 10^9/l$)
Lymphocytes	$1.97 \times 10^9/l$ (normal $1.5-4.0 \times 10^9/l$)
Monocytes	$0.48 \times 10^9/l$ (normal $0.3-0.8 \times 10^9/l$)
Eosinophils	$1.05 \times 10^9/l$ (normal $0.04-0.4 \times 10^9/l$)
Basophils	$0.02 \times 10^9/l$ (normal $0.01-0.1 \times 10^9/l$)

IgG antibodies against gliadin are positive in her blood but IgA antibodies are negative. Jejunal biospy shows villous atrophy.

1. What is the most likely diagnosis?

Question 6.9

A 6-month-old infant is admitted because of failure to thrive. Investigations give the following results:

Plasma sodium	140 mmol/l
Plasma potassium	3.0 mmol/l
Plasma urea	5 mmol/l
Plasma chloride	115 mmol/l
Plasma glucose	4 mmol/l
Arterial blood gases:	
pH	7.3
PaO_2	12 kPa
$PaCO_2$	3.7 kPa
Bicarbonate	15 mmol/l

The urine was positive on testing for glucose but free of casts, white and red cells on microscopy. Urine pH = 6.

1. What is the diagnosis?

Question 6.10

An 8-year-old child presents with muscle weakness. Blood pressure is 150 mmHg systolic, 105 mmHg diastolic. The following blood results are obtained from a venous sample:

Plasma potassium	2.9 mmol/l ↓
pH	7.5 ↑
$PaCO_2$	6.1 kPa
PaO_2	5.2 kPa
Bicarbonate	30 mmol/l
Plasma renin	Decreased
Plasma cortisol	Normal

1. What is the diagnosis?
2. Suggest two tests on a urine sample which would help confirm this diagnosis.

Paper 6 ANSWERS

Answer 6.1

1. Hypsarrhythmia
2. Infantile spasms

Discussion

The term hypsarrhythmia is used to describe the EEG pattern commonly associated with infantile spasms. The pattern consists of high voltage, arrhythmic slow waves interspersed with spiked discharges showing multifocal distribution. Hypsarrhythmia refers only to the EEG pattern and should not be used to describe the clinical condition. Hypsarrhythmia usually appears around 6 months and is rare before 3 months, tending to disappear or modify after 12 months of age. The hypsarrhythmic pattern may be enhanced by drowsiness and sleep, especially in the early phases and during the course of treatment.

In infantile spasms, the onset of attacks is in the first year of life in 90% of cases, and in the first 6 months in nearly 70%, with a peak incidence at about 5 months. There is sudden brief flexion of neck and trunk, raising of both arms forwards or sideways, sometimes with flexion at the elbows and flexion of the legs at the hips. Less often the legs extend at the hips. A cry is often associated with the attacks and may form part of the attack or occur afterwards as an expression of distress.

The importance of the syndrome lies in its close association with mental retardation. It is usual for the onset of spasms to be followed quickly by slowing down in the infant's development and often by marked regression, with loss of acquired skills and social responsiveness. In untreated, and many treated, persisting cases severe mental retardation is very common. Spasms usually cease by the age of 2 years but are often followed by major convulsions.

Treatment with conventional anticonvulsants gives disappointing results. Benzodiazepines abolish or reduce attacks and sometimes improve the EEG. However, the ultimate prognosis for intelligence rarely seems to be improved by these. Sodium valproate has given good results in some cases. ACTH and oral steroid preparations were introduced on the suspicion of an underlying neuro-allergic encephalitis. Although this is unlikely, good results were obtained and this approach is the most successful one available.

Further reading
Brett E (ed) 1991 Paediatric neurology, 2nd edn. Churchill Livingstone, Edinburgh, pp. 325–330

Answer 6.2

1. Reinforcing dose of adsorbed toxoid vaccine plus a dose of human anti-tetanus toxin immunoglobulin

Discussion

Contamination of a wound with stable manure puts the patient into a high-risk group for developing tetanus. It is important to remember that thorough surgical toilet of the wound is essential whatever the immunization status of the patient. The following wounds should be considered tetanus prone:

— any wound or burn sustained >6 h before surgical treatment;
— any wound or burn at any interval after injury that shows one or more of the following characteristics: a significant degree of devitalized tissue, puncture-type wound, contact with soil or manure likely to harbour tetanus organisms, clinical evidence of sepsis.

Specific anti-tetanus prophylaxis

Immunization status	Wound clean	Tetanus-prone wound
Last of 3 dose course, or reinforcing dose within last 10 years	Nil	Nil (dose of adsorbed vaccine may be given if risk of infection is considered especially high, e.g. contamination with stable manure)
Last of 3 dose course or reinfrocing dose 10 years ago	Reinforcing dose of adsorbed vaccine	Reinforcing dose of adsorbed vaccine plus dose of human tetanus immunoglobulin
Not immunized or status not known with certainty	Full 3 dose course adsorbed vaccine	Full 3 dose course of vaccine, plus dose of tetanus immunoglobulin in a different site

Answer 6.3

1. Supraventricular tachycardia
2. Adenosine
   Cardioversion
   Vagal stimulation

Discussion

This child has a supraventricular tachycardia. It is not a sinus tachycardia because the rate of 300 beats/min is too fast; in sinus tachycardia it does not exceed 210 beats/min. It is differentiated from ventricular tachycardia in as far as the QRS duration is of normal length.

Paroxysmal supraventricular tachycardia may present as a true medical emergency in infancy. When prolonged it may result in severe peripheral and central circulatory failure and urgent treatment is necessary. Adenosine is *is*

effective and the treatment of choice. It acts by preventing passage of electrical impulses through the atrioventricular node. This may stop the episode if there is a reciprocating tachycardia, and slows the ventricular rate revealing the underlying atrial rhythm in atrial fibrillation or flutter. Its half life is only a matter of seconds.

If adenosine is unavailable or unsuccessful after repeated doses, cardioversion is the next line treatment. Cardioversion should be with a synchronized defibrillator with levels of 0.5–1.0 W/s/kg.

For less acutely ill infants, vagal manoeuvres can be attempted. The diving reflex is the most successful and is best elicited by covering the infant's face with a small plastic bag filled with ice or immersing the infant's face in ice-cold water for a few seconds.

Answer 6.4

1. The results are normal

Discussion

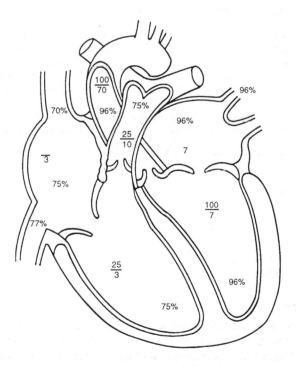

An idea of normality allows assessment of other cardiac catheter results. The figure above illustrates both blood pressure and oxygen saturation in the various chambers and vessels involved. Diagnostic cardiac catheterization and angiocardiography are undertaken to obtain detailed information on the anatomical abnormality and its haemodynamic effects, such as pressure gradients, pulmonary artery pressure, shunt size and pulmonary vascular resistance. Catheterization is increasingly undertaken, not for diagnostic purposes but for treatment. Balloon dilatation of the pulmonary valve is an accepted technique, but dilatation for aortic stenosis and coarctation of the aorta are still not universally accepted. Closure of an arterial duct is gaining acceptability and it is possible that in the future closure of ventricular or atrial septal defects may become the treatment of choice in certain patients.

The oxygen saturation is usually measured in the large veins, atria, ventricles and great arteries. A significant left-to-right shunt is suggested by a rise in oxygen saturation of 5% or more in the right atrium (atrial septal defects), right ventricle (ventricular septal defect) or pulmonary artery (ductus arteriosus). The arterial oxygen saturation gives an estimate of the severity of, and the need for intervention surgically, in cyanotic congenital heart disease.

Pressures are measured in the atria, ventricles and great arteries. Mean pressure in the atria and great arteries is required for estimation of pulmonary or systemic vascular resistance and peak points in the ventricles and arteries for measuring transvalve gradient. In children, the simple valve gradient rather than valve area is generally used to determine the need for surgical intervention. The pulmonary vascular resistance, rather than the pulmonary artery pressure, is the main determinant of the prognosis and indeed the operability of a child with a left-to-right shunt. Where it is elevated, it is appropriate to assess whether it is fixed or can be reduced by the administration of a pulmonary vasodilator such as 100% oxygen or tolazoline.

Selective cine angiography or digital subtraction angiography is performed by the injection of radiological contrast into the chamber or vessel immediately proximal to the abnormality. With the advent of ultrasound, angiocardiography is now less important for the diagnosis of intracardiac defects, but it remains necessary for abnormalities of the great arteries or veins, in particular the anatomy of the pulmonary artery and its branches in situations where they are reduced in size.

Although cardiac catheterization is usually a safe procedure, death can occur, most commonly in those with severe pulmonary hypertension. Complications include femoral artery occlusion, dysrhythmias, intramyocardial injection with pericardial effusion, cerebral embolus and cerebral thrombosis.

Answer 6.5

1. Hypochromic microcytic anaemia
2. Iron-deficiency anaemia
3. Small red cells (microcytes) and pale (hypochromic) red cells. Elliptical and elongated pencil cells and cells of differing sizes (anisocytosis) are often seen

Discussion

Iron-deficiency anaemia is relatively common in childhood. Causes are usually multifactorial and include age, diet, ethnic background and economic status. Up to 20% of cases with iron deficiency have a normal blood film and occasionally the blood film from a normal child may show morphological features suggestive of iron deficiency. Thomobocytosis, in association with iron deficiency, may indicate chronic blood loss, usually gastrointestinal.

Serum ferritin is proportional to the levels of storage iron and is a sensitive and reproducible quantitative assay of body iron stores. Serum ferritin helps to differentiate between iron deficiency and the anaemia of chronic disorders. In iron-deficiency anaemia, ferritin is low. In anaemia due to chronic disease, the serum ferritin is raised, whilst in thalassaemia minor it is normal. In acute and chronic leukaemia, hepatic failure and some other malignancies, serum ferritin may not be a true reflection of body iron stores.

In iron-deficiency anaemia, the serum iron level is usually reduced and the iron-binding capacity raised. However, both are subject to large variations depending on sex, age, laboratory methods, diurnal variation and diet.

Further reading

Campbell A G M, McIntosh N (eds) 1992 Forfar and Arneil's Textbook of paediatrics, 4th edn. Churchill Livingstone, Edinburgh, pp. 1281–1282

Answer 6.6

1. Yes
2. Confirms transplacental blood loss

Discussion

Anaemia due to blood loss is more common during the newborn period than at any time throughout childhood. Acute haemorrhage of >20–30% of the infant's blood volume results in the signs and symptoms of shock. These include pallor, lethargy, tachycardia and hypotension.

A positive Kleihauer test confirms transplacental haemorrhage from the fetus to the mother. As both the fetal and maternal ABO and Rh blood groups are identical and the Coombs' test negative, isoimmune haemolytic disease is very unlikely.

Fetal red cells containing HbF can be identified by the Kleihauer test as they are more resistant to acid elution than maternal cells. Maternal blood is taken to prepare blood films which are subjected to acid elution and stained. The fetal cells stain red and adult cells pink.

Certain limitations are attached to the Kleihauer test. For example, ABO incompatibility between mother and baby may result in rapid elimination of fetal cells, and up to 10% of fetal cells do not contain HbF or stain typically. In addition, conditions such as sickle cell anaemia, or thalassaemia minor, may result in an elevated HbF level.

Answer 6.7

1. Chronic obstructive sleep apnoea
2. Overnight pulse oximetry
   Overnight monitoring of arterial blood gases
   Indirect laryngoscopy
   Electrocardiogram

   Echocardiogram

Discussion

There is hypercapnia during the night and a compensatory metabolic alkalosis is obvious on both blood gases. The most likely diagnosis is chronic obstructive sleep apnoea and if all the arterial blood gas data had been given, these would show nocturnal hypoxia in addition to hypercapnia.

Upper airways obstruction becomes critical during sleep. Symptoms usually develop from the age of 2 years onwards, but can also be seen in infancy, and may be severe enough to cause failure to thrive. The parents often describe a child who is a mouth breather by day and a very restless, noisy sleeper by night. The child is often reported to snore loudly. He may be more irritable in the morning, because his sleep has been interrupted, and sleepy throughout the day; an older child may complain of morning headaches (due to CO_2 retention overnight) or poor school performance.

Upper airways obstruction with snoring is usually caused by enlarged tonsils and adenoids but may also occur due to mandibular or maxillary malformation, deviation of the nasal septum, enlarged tongue, congenital laryngeal anomalies, vocal cord paralysis (the cords adopt the adducted position following tenth nerve palsy) or severe obesity. It is particularly common in Down's syndrome. Apart from the upper airways obstruction, any cause of nocturnal hypoventilation could produce a similar pattern of blood gases, e.g. severe kyphoscoliosis, a myopathy affecting the intercostal muscles or diaphragm, or congenital central hypoventilation (Ondine's curse).

The diagnosis is confirmed by overnight pulse oximetry which is non-invasive. If accompanied by monitoring of nasal airflow (e.g. by a nasal thermistor), periods of desaturation can be seen to follow episodes of decreased or absent airflow. If arterial blood gases are used to make the diagnosis, an indwelling arterial catheter is essential so that the sampling of blood does not alert the child.

Indirect laryngoscopy will usually confirm the need for tonsillectomy alone or with adenoidectomy. Symptoms resolve rapidly and a growth spurt often follows surgery.

An electrocardiogram should be done to look for peaked P waves (>3 mm suggests 'P pulmonale') and voltage changes of right ventricular hypertrophy, both of which imply the development of pulmonary hypertension. Chronic hypoxia is a potent cause of hypertrophy of the pulmonary arterioles and chronic obstructive sleep apnoea may be sufficiently severe to cause cor pulmonale. Electrocardiography is more sensitive at detecting ventricular hypertrophy than echocardiography.

Further reading
Anon 1992 Snoring children, sleep apnoea and tonsillectomy. Drug and Therapeutics Bulletin 30(2): 6–7
Stradling J R, Thomas G, Warley A R H, Williams P, Freeland A 1990 Effect of adenotonsillectomy on nocturnal hypoxaemia, sleep disturbance, and symptoms in snoring children. Lancet 335: 249–253

Answer 6.8

1. Cows' milk protein intolerance

Malabsorption due to small bowel disease
Post-gastroenteritis malabsorption
Failure to thrive due to small bowel disease

Discussion

The child's weight is below the 3rd centile but she is receiving adequate intake of milk (approx. 150 ml/kg/day). Cows' milk protein intolerance most commonly develops within the first 6 months of life, whereas in coeliac disease the majority develop symptoms between 9 months and 2 years of age, following the onset of weaning and the introduction of solid foods containing wheat, barley or rye, all of which contain gluten. The most common symptoms in cows' milk protein intolerance are vomiting, diarrhoea and poor weight gain. Eczema is frequently present in the index case at presentation and there may be a history of atopy in the family, which may include asthma or hayfever in older children. The eosinophilia shown in the blood count is characteristic of cows' milk protein intolerance and serum immunoglobulins may also show a non-specifically raised IgE level, although both of these abnormalities are non-specific. The haemoglobin of 9.4 g/dl is not abnormally low for a child of this age.

Villous atrophy on jejunal biopsy is not diagnostic of coeliac disease and other causes of this include transient gluten intolerance, cows' milk protein intolerance, soy protein intolerance, and following gastroenteritis. Less common causes are giardiasis, severe combined immunodeficiency syndrome and following cytotoxic chemotherapy.

IgG antibodies against gliadin are positive in 98% of children with coeliac disease but also in 30% of other gastrointestinal disorders. This test is therefore sensitive but not specific. The presence of IgA antibodies against gliadin is a more specific investigation in that it is positive in 77% of children who have coeliac disease but only in 3% who do not. This test is therefore less sensitive. The level of antibody against IgA also declines within weeks of starting a gluten-free diet and this may be used to monitor response and compliance.

To be certain of a diagnosis of coeliac disease requires the combination of the appropriate clinical picture, villous atrophy on jejunal biopsy, clinical and histological response to gluten withdrawal from the diet, and proof of clinical or histological relapse on rechallenge with gluten. Until recently, only this third biopsy allowed the distinction between coeliac disease, which is permanent and carries a long-term risk of intestinal neoplasm, and transient gluten intolerance, which does not require a strict lifelong diet. However, the advent of immunological tests for gluten-sensitive enteropathy and for monitoring the response to a gluten-free diet may, in the future, allow this third biopsy to be withdrawn from the protocol.

Further reading

Campbell A G M, McIntosh N (eds) 1992 Forfar and Arneil's Textbook of paediatrics, 4th edn. Churchill Livingstone, Edinburgh, pp. 507–511
Walker-Smith J A 1975 Cow's milk protein intolerance: transient food intolerance of infancy. Archives of Disease in Childhood 50: 346–350

Answer 6.9

1. Proximal renal tubular acidosis

Discussion

There is a metabolic acidosis with respiratory compensation and hence a low $PaCO_2$. The metabolic acidosis is accompanied by a normal anion gap (anion gap is the plasma sodium concentration minus the combined chloride and bicarbonate concentration and is normally 9–30 mmol/l). There is glycosuria despite a normal blood glucose but no evidence from the blood or urine results of either renal failure or parenchymal renal damage. The combination of metabolic acidosis with a normal anion gap and renal glycosuria is highly suggestive of proximal renal tubular acidosis.

The normal anion gap is 9–30 mmol/l because the sodium concentration normally exceeds the combined chloride and bicarbonate concentration. This is because the circulating plasma proteins predominantly have a negative charge and this constitutes most of this anion gap. Determining the anion gap is helpful in the differential diagnosis of a child with metabolic acidosis.

Gastrointestinal or renal loss of bicarbonate produces a hyperchloraemic acidosis because the fall in plasma bicarbonate concentration is mirrored by a parallel increase in plasma chloride concentration, such that the anion gap remains constant. This is because the kidney retains chloride in an effort to preserve the circulating volume which would be depleted if electrical balance were maintained instead by sodium being lost with bicarbonate. On the other hand, if the acidosis is the result of hydrogen ions accumulating with another anion, rather than loss of bicarbonate, then this anion (e.g. lactate or ketoacids) will increase the anion gap. It must be emphasized however, that the calculation of the anion gap is merely a help in the differential diagnosis. Whatever the size of the anion gap, it is the retention of hydrogen ions and not of any particular anion that is responsible for the acidosis.

Approximately 90% of bicarbonate reabsorption occurs in the proximal tubule. In patients with proximal renal tubular acidosis there is a reduction in proximal tubular bicarbonate reabsorption resulting in bicarbonate loss in the urine and a metabolic acidosis. This is usually a self-limiting disorder since as the plasma bicarbonate concentration falls, the amount of bicarbonate filtered also falls. The bicarbonate wasting ceases when the filtered bicarbonate load falls and this usually occurs when the plasma bicarbonate concentration reaches 15–20 mmol/l. Plasma bicarbonate concentrations below 15–20 mmol/l are therefore rarely seen as a feature of proximal renal tubular acidosis. In addition to the defect in bicarbonate reabsorption, a variety of other proximal functions may be impaired, such as the reabsorption of phosphate, uric acid, amino acids and glucose.

The correction of acidosis is difficult since any bicarbonate administered is excreted in the urine and to stay ahead of renal excretion requires massive amounts of bicarbonate supplement, averaging 10–15 mmol/kg/day.

Children with *distal* renal tubular acidosis can present with failure to thrive and weakness but unlike proximal acidosis, there is no glycosuria or generalized aminoaciduria. In distal tubular acidosis there may be nephrocalicinosis due to hypercalcuria.

In the distal condition, bicarbonate reabsorption is normal but there is impaired ability to secrete hydrogen ion into the distal tubules and urine pH cannot be lowered below 5.5 (normal urine pH 4.5–5.0). Unlike proximal tubular acidosis, the distal renal tubular acidosis is progressive rather than self-limiting since hydrogen ions are retained every day. However, treatment with bicarbonate supplements is easier as the amount of bicarbonate required will not exceed the daily hydrogen load of 2–3 mmol/kg/day in children. Bicarbonate is effective in treating distal renal tubular acidosis, because the bicarbonate appearing in the urine acts as a buffer and allows hydrogen ion secretion in the distal nephron to continue without reaching the lower limiting urine pH of 5.5.

In the absence of an infection with a urea splitting organism (which elevates the urine pH. e.g proteus), only proximal and distal renal tubular acidosis can produce a metabolic acidosis in blood with a urine pH >5.3.

Distal and proximal renal tubular acidosis can be distinguished by either bicarbonate loading (in proximal renal tubular acidosis the urine becomes more alkaline whereas in distal renal tubular acidosis the urine pH is unchanged) or by ammonium chloride loading (in proximal renal tubular acidosis the urine becomes more acidic whereas in distal renal tubular acidosis the pH remains unchanged).

The renal tubular acidoses are sometimes confused with two other disorders. Bartter's syndrome is a failure of proximal tubular reabsorption of chloride and therefore also of sodium. The outcome is hyponatraemia, profound hypokalaemia with metabolic acidosis, polyuria and activation of the renin angiotensin system. In hypoaldosteronism, there is a failure of the distal tubule to exchange hydrogen ions or potassium for sodium and therefore there is hyponatraemia and hyperkalaemia with metabolic acidosis.

Answer 6.10

1. Primary hyperaldosteronism
2. Urinary sodium:potassium ratio
   Urinary aldosterone metabolites

   Urine steroid screen (or some other non-specific phrase)

Discussion

This child shows the classical features of hypertension due to sodium retention with hypokalaemic alkalosis. The fact that there is also renin suppression demonstrates that this must be primary hyperaldosterinism (Conn's syndrome). In secondary hyperaldosteronism (e.g. due to hypovolaemia due to diuretic abuse or ascites or due to decreased renal blood flow from renal artery stenosis) the renin concentration will be high and drives secretion of aldosterone. The normal cortisol level excludes Cushing's syndrome which is a far commoner cause of hyperadrenalism in childhood, most frequently iatrogenic (oral steroids used for chronic renal disease, tumours, immunosuppression, connective tissue disorders and asthma, or ACTH used to treat hypsarrhythmia).

Primary hyperaldosteronism is a rare condition in childhood, due to an aldosterone-secreting adenoma (80%) or to diffuse adrenocorticol hyperplasia, or more rarely a carcinoma of the adrenal cortex. Aldosterone causes sodium reabsorption in exchange for potassium and hydrogen ions in the distal tubules of the kidney. Diagnosis is suspected by the combination of hypertension and hypokalaemia but 20% of patients will have normal potassium levels at presentation. However, these potassium levels will fall below the normal range following administration of oral sodium. Muscle weakness is due to hypokalaemia and the children may also present with polyuria or nocturnal enuresis.

The action of aldosterone in the distal tubule will result in a decreased ratio of sodium to potassium in urine (as a rough guide there is usually about twice as much sodium as potassium in urine expressed as mmol/kg/24 h). The second investigation would be to demonstrate high levels of urinary aldosterone metabolites.

Hypernatraemia is a less common finding than hyponatraemia in childhood and is most commonly caused by sodium overload either by the parents making concentrated feeds or by doctors administering hypertonic intravenous solutions. Water depletion can also lead to hypernatraemia, and is seen following excessive transepidermal water loss in the newborn, and with excessive renal water loss in diabetes insipidus. In the neonatal period, hypernatraemia is more commonly due to water depletion, in contrast to older children.

Further reading

Campbell A G M, McIntosh N (eds) 1992 Forfar and Arneil's Textbook of paediatrics, 4th edn. Churchill Livingstone, Edinburgh, p. 163, 475
De Swiet M, Dillon M J 1989 Hypertension in children. British Medical Journal 299: 465–470

Paper 7 *QUESTIONS*

Question 7.1

Concerns were raised over the hearing of an 8-year-old boy. Rinne and Weber tests were performed. In the right ear, he was Rinne positive, but the Weber test was to the right. In the left ear he was Rinne negative.

1. What is your interpretation of these results?

Question 7.2

This is the ECG trace from an 8-year-old boy.

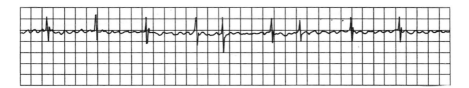

1. What does the ECG trace show?

Question 7.3

These are the blood pressure readings from three children:

Mary (4 years)	120/95 mmHg
John (1 month)	65/45 mmHg
Christopher (1 year)	115/90 mmHg

1. Which of these children require(s) follow up for blood pressure measurements?

Question 7.4

A 10-year-old boy presented with discomfort of his hands and feet and severe lightning pains in his arms and legs which were aggravated by exercise. Examination revealed a cluster of red papules on his skin that did not fade on pressure. Urine showed an abnormal level of ceramide trihexoside.

1. What is the most likely diagnosis?

Question 7.5

A 12-year-old boy with Fallot's tetralogy is admitted with right hemiplegia.

Platelet count	$100 \times 10^9/l$
Haemoglobin	17.0 g/dl
White cell count	$13 \times 10^9/l$
Polymorphs	80%

1. What are the two most likely diagnoses?
2. What further investigation is required?

Question 7.6

A baby girl was noted to have radial deviation of her hands at birth, short forearms and widespread purpura. Investigation results were:

Haemoglobin	17 g/dl
White cell count	$20 \times 10^9/l$
Platelet count	$17 \times 10^9/l$
Bone marrow	Small, abnormal megakaryocytes
TORCH screen	Negative
Chromosomal analysis	Normal

1. What is the most likely diagnosis?
2. What investigation would help confirm your diagnosis?

Question 7.7

A well 4-kg male infant was noted to vomit blood 12 h after delivery. The following results were obtained:

Haemoglobin	14 g/dl
Prothrombin time	12 s (control 12 s)
Thrombin time	16 s (control 16 s)
Partial thromboplastin time	40 s (control 40 s)
Apt test	Positive (yellow–brown colour)

1. What is the most likely cause of his blood-stained vomit?

Question 7.8

A 3-year-old boy is investigated for steatorrhoea and failure to thrive.

Haemoglobin	12.0 g/dl
White cell count	$3.8 \times 10^9/l$
Neutrophils	23%
Platelet count	$88 \times 10^9/l$
Faecal fats	Markedly raised
Jejunal biopsy	Normal
Sweat test	Normal

1. What is the most likely diagnosis?
2. What is the explanation for the haematological values?

Question 7.9

A 10-year-old child was investigated for renal colic. The amino acids arginine, lysine, cystine and ornithine were found on amino acid chromatography of his urine.

1. What is the diagnosis?
2. What three other clinical problems may occur in this condition?

Question 7.10

The following blood and urine results were obtained from a child:

Urine volume	5 litres in 24 h
Urine specific gravity	1.003
Plasma osmolality	290 mOsmol/kg H_2O
Plasma urea	4.5 mmol/l
Urine osmolality	150 mOsmol/kg H_2O
Urine glucose	Negative
Urine protein on dipstick testing	Negative

1. What three diagnoses could explain these data?
2. What two tests would distinguish them?

Paper 7 *Answers*

Answer 7.1

1. Left-sided severe or profound sensorineural hearing loss

Discussion

In the Rinne test, the patient's ability to discriminate between air conduction and bone conduction is tested. To test air conduction the tines of the fork are held parallel to the ear canal and about 1" away. For bone conduction testing the base of the fork is held firmly against the skull adjacent to the ear, typically against the mastoid process. The patient is asked to compare the loudness of the bone-conducted and air-conducted sound. A positive Rinne test is recorded when air conduction is heard better than bone conduction, and negative when the converse is found.

In the Weber's test, the tuning fork is held on the vertex of the skull in the midline and the patient is asked whether he can hear the sound and if so whether it lateralizes.

Right	Left	Interpretation
Rinne positive/Weber central	Rinne positive	Normal/mild or severe bilateral sensorineural loss
Rinne positive/Weber to left	Rinne negative	Left conductive or mixed hearing loss
Rinne negative/Weber central	Rinne negative	Bilateral mixed or conductive deafness
Rinne positive/Weber to right	Rinne negative	Left severe or profound sensorineural loss

Answer 7.2

1. Atrial fibrillation

Discussion

Atrial flutter and fibrillation are uncommon arrhythmias in children and often result from long-standing heart disease. They can complicate myocardial disease and mitral valve disease. In atrial flutter there is an atrial rate of 280 beats/min or greater. The ventricles may only respond intermittently at ratios of 2:1–4:1. In atrial fibrillation the atrial activity is totally disordered and the ventricular response irregular.

Answer 7.3

1. Mary and Christopher

Discussion

It is important to know, or have access to, centile charts for blood pressure readings in childhood (see Report on the 2nd Task Force on Blood Pressure in Children 1987). It has been suggested that levels >95th centile for age should be considered abnormal, and on this basis supine blood pressure values above the following should be regarded as indicating significant hypertension:

1 week–1 month	104 mmHg systolic
1 month–1 year	112/74 mmHg
3–5 years	116/76 mmHg
6–9 years	112/78 mmHg
10–12 years	126/82 mmHg
13–15 years	136/86 mmHg
16–18 years	142/92 mmHg

Blood pressure should be measured with the child lying or sitting comfortably with the sphygmomanometer at heart level. The cuff must cover at least two-thirds of the upper arm. Narrower cuffs give falsely high results. Blood pressure in children is labile and a single reading cannot be considered to indicate hypertension unless it is very high. The reading should be repeated, and only if the level has been found to be elevated on at least three occasions can the patient be considered to have hypertension.

Hypertension is increasingly recognized in paediatric practice. Sustained hypertension is significant and always requires investigation. Primary (essential) hypertension is rare in children with severe hypertension but is fairly common in those with mild or borderline hypertension. Coarctation of the aorta is the commonest cause in infants under 1 year of age. Beyond infancy, renal disorders explain more than 80% of cases

Causes of sustained hypertension:

Cardiovascular:	Coarctation of the aorta
Renal:	Chronic renal failure
	Renin dependent hypertension
	Renovascular disease
	Renal tumours
Catecholamine excess:	Neuroblastoma
	Phaochromocytoma
Corticosteroid excess:	Iatrogenic
	Congenital adrenal hyperplasia
	Conn's syndrome
	Cushing's syndrome

Further reading
 Report on the 2nd Task Force on Blood Pressure in Children 1987
 Pediatrics 79: 1–25

Answer 7.4

1. Fabry's disease

Discussion

Fabry's disease is characterized by abnormal accumulation of ceramide trihexoside in the vascular endothelium. It is sex-linked with onset of symptoms around puberty. There may be gastrointestinal symptoms, distal parasthesia and fever crises. Clusters of dark red to blue black punctate lesions, often in the 'bathing trunk' distribution, may be noticed in childhood. Eye changes, including aneurysmal dilatation of vessels in the conjunctiva and retina may occur. The disease can present as renal failure, a cerebrovascular accident, or with tetangiectasia of the sclera or skin. Death usually occurs in the fourth decade.

In Fabry's disease there is deficient α-galactosidase A activity leading to the abnormal accumulation of ceramide trihexoside. Enzyme diagnosis is carried out on plasma, leucocytes or cultured fibroblasts. Antenatal screening tests for heterozygotes are available. *(deficiency of α-galactosidase activity in cultured chorionic villi or amniocytes)*

Futher reading
 Brett E M 1991 *Paediatric neurology,* 2nd edn. Churchill Livingstone,
 Edinburgh, pp. 158–159.

Answer 7.5

1. Cerebral abscess
 Cerebral infarction
 Cerebral thrombosis
2. Brain CT with contrast enhancement

 Brain CT
 Brain MRI scan

Discussion

A cerebral abscess must always be considered in a child with right-to-left cardiac shunt who presents with focal neurological signs. A CT head scan with contrast enhancement must be obtained quickly. If this shows no abscess (this should appear as a focal mass lesion with ring enhancement following contrast injection) or just an area of infarction, the most likely diagnosis would be polycythaemic cerebral arterial or dural sinus thrombosis. Treatment of the cerebral abscess is usually by excision, drainage and antibiotics. MRI scan of the brain will show focal lesions but this investigation is less readily available and scores fewer marks.

Some increase in the haematocrit in this boy is beneficial as the oxygen carrying capacity of the blood is increased. There will be an increase in total blood volume due to the increased red cell mass. Plasma volume is normal or reduced. It has been shown that at any given haematocrit, cardiac output is greater with hypervolaemia than with normovolaemia provided cardiac function is reasonable. Clearly this is not true when there is overt cardiac failure. If the haematocrit becomes too high, however, this benefit is lost and the sudden increase in viscosity increases the risk of a cerebrovascular accident. Children with polycythaemia secondary to congenital heart disease, combined with iron deficiency (microcytic hypochromia cells), seem to be at greatest risk of cerebral infarction.

The haematocrit may be reduced by exchanging plasma for blood, thus maintaining the hypervolaemia but reducing the blood viscosity. As a result there will be an increase in cerebral blood flow. An exchange transfusion should start by giving plasma rather than withdrawal of blood as the combination of hypovolaemia and hyperviscosity can seriously compromise cerebral blood flow further. One of the benefits of corrective cardiac surgery in early life for tetralogy of Fallot is to avoid this kind of complication in later childhood. Before further surgery is considered on this boy, it would be necessary by cardiac catheter or ultrasound studies to demonstrate that he had not developed Eisenmenger's syndrome (suprasystemic pressures on the right side of the heart), which precludes further surgery.

Answer 7.6

1. Thrombocytopenia with absent radii syndrome
2. Skeletal survey to confirm bilateral radial aplasia

Discussion

Thrombocytopenia with absent radii syndrome is usually recognized at birth and is an isolated failure of platelet production. There are no associated chromosomal abnormalities. The white blood cell count is often increased with a leukamoid reaction in addition to significant thrombocytopenia. The raised white cell count usually improves with time, though thrombocytopenia persists. The survival of transfused platelets is normal. With good cross-matching of platelets, many patients can be maintained, if necessary, on weekly platelet transfusions for long periods of time. Bleeding tendency and platelet count do, however, improve with age.

Answer 7.7

1. Swallowed maternal blood

Discussion

In the newborn period when haematemesis or melena occur, the question as to whether this represents swallowed maternal blood or blood from the baby is addressed by performing the Apt test for fetal haemoglobin. The Apt differentiates fetal and adult (maternal) haemoglobin in stool or vomitus — if the solution remains pink, HbF is present; if it turns yellow–brown, HbA (maternal blood) is present.

Answer 7.8

1. Schwachman's syndrome
2. Myeloid series arrest

   Arrest of white cell and platelet production

Discussion

There is malabsorption with neutropenia (absolute neutrophil count $<1.0 \times 10^9/l$). Apart from cystic fibrosis, Schwachman's syndrome (or Schwachman-Diamond syndrome) is the commonest cause of failure of the exocrine pancreas and is associated with neutropenia, which may be cyclical, and a neutrophil chemotactic defect. Cyclical thrombocytopenia occurs in two-thirds of cases. Other findings are short stature, metaphyseal chondrodysplasia on limb X-rays and sometimes hepatomegaly. Although usually sporadic, autosomal recessive inheritance has been reported.

Arrest in proliferation of the myeloid series is seen on bone marrow aspiration.

Further reading

Aggett P J, Cavanach N P C, Mathew D J, Pincott J R, Sutcliffe J, Harries J T 1980 Schwachman's syndrome. Archives of Disease in Childhood 55: 331–347

Milner A D, Hull D 1992 Hospital paediatrics, 2nd edn. Churchill Livingstone, Edinburgh, p. 149.

Answer 7.9

1. Cystinuria
2. Haematuria
   Obstruction to urine flow and secondary pyelonephritis
   Renal failure

Discussion

Cystinuria is a disorder of intestinal absorption and renal tubular reabsorption of the dibasic amino acids arginine, lysine, cystine and orthinine. Although dibasic amino acid absorption is reduced due to a transport defect in the intestinal mucosa, they can be synthesized in the body, and deficiency does not occur. The incidence is about 1 in 650 of the population but only 3% of affected individuals form calculi.   *magenta-red* ←

The nitroprusside test will detect large amounts of cystine in the urine, and the typical amino acid excretory pattern is confirmed by chromatography.

There are at least three types of genetic abnormalities in the group transport of cystine and the dibasic amino acids in the gut and kidney. Urinary amino acid levels are the same in all types of homozygotes. Heterozygotes for type 1 have no aminociduria but heterozygotes for types 2 and 3 may have sufficient cystinuria and lysinuria to cause calculus formation.

The clinical importance of cystinuria lies in the risk of calculi formation which may cause haematuria, obstruction to urine flow, secondary pyelonephritis and renal failure. Prevention of recurrence following surgical removal of calculi and prevention of calculi formation in asymptomatic family members are of importance. Treatment includes: water diuresis, alkalinization of urine with sodium citrate or bicarbonate, or D-penicillamine on a semi-permanent basis.

Further reading

Campbell A G M, McIntosh N (eds) 1992 Forfar and Arneil's Textbook of paediatrics, 4th edn. Churchill Livingstone, Edinburgh, pp. 1026–1194

Answer 7.10

1. Psychogenic polydipsia
   Central diabetes insipidus
   Nephrogenic diabetes insipidus
2. Water deprivation test
   Desamino-8-D-arginine vasopressin (DDAVP) challenge

   Hypotonic saline infusion

Discussion

The child has either psychogenic polydipsia or diabetes insipidus, which may be central or nephrogenic. The candidate cannot distinguish between these causes from the data provided.

Serum osmolality is normally between 285 and 295 mmol/kg H_2O. The child has polyuria, which is very hypotonic (average urine output is 0.5 l/day at 1 year of age, 1 l/day at 8 years and 1.5 l/day at 15 years), and a normal plasma osmolality. Urine specific gravity and osmolality are unreliable in the presence of glycosuria or significant proteinuria but neither of these are present. Beyond the neonatal period, the child can produce urine with a range between 30 mOsmol/kg H_2O and 1200 mOsmol/kg. Osmolality has a non-linear relationship with specific gravity. Thirty mOsmol/l corresponds to a specific gravity of about 1.000, 300 mOsmol/kg to 1.010 and 500 mOsmol/kg to 1.022. As the plasma is not hypertonic, the very high daily urine output must be accompanied by high daily fluid intake. Possible explanations are either that the child is voluntarily drinking a great deal, causing a large output of hypotonic urine as an appropriate homeostatic response *or* the child has a large obligatory renal water loss and drinking is driven by a thirst mechanism to keep pace with this.

Compulsive water drinking can be distinguished from diabetes insipidus by a water deprivation test. In psychogenic polydipsia, the urine osmolality will rise appropriately above plasma osmolality following water deprivation. Confusion may arise, however, because prolonged compulsive water drinking can reduce the ability of the kidney to concentrate urine and there can be an impaired response, even to exogenous DDAVP (desamino-8-D-arginine vasopressin, an analogue of natural arginine vasopressin). A water deprivation test which lasts for 8–12 h and involves at least a loss of 3% body weight may be hazardous, particularly in a young infant or one in whom the plasma osmolality is already raised. Such fluid deprivation may lead to rapid weight loss with hypernatraemia, hypovolaemia and haemoconcentration.

Central and nephrogenic diabetes insipidus may be distinguished by giving DDAVP intravenously or intranasally. This is immediately followed by a large reduction in urine volume in the case of central diabetes insipidus. In nephrogenic diabetes insipidus there is end-organ insensitivity to antidiuretic hormone and therefore no response to a DDAVP test. Central diabetes insipidus is most commonly due to damage to the posterior pituitary lobe either by trauma, pituitary surgery, histiocytosis X, sarcoidosis, encephalitis or by a tumour such as a craniopharyngioma. Visual fields should be tested (looking for evidence of pressure on the optic chiasma) and a CT scan arranged. Nephrogenic diabetes insipidus may be inherited in a sex-linked fashion. Polyuria and reduced concentrating ability are also features of chronic renal failure or a tubular defect but the normal plasma urea and the absence of glycosuria and proteinuria are against these diagnoses.

A third diagnostic test is the infusion of hypertonic saline. The normal child produces a reduced volume of urine of increased osmolality, whereas no change in urine flow rate is seen in central or nephrogenic diabetes insipidus. This is a potentially dangerous test which is rarely done.

Further reading

Hughes I A 1989 Handbook of endocrine investigations in children. John Wright, Bristol

Perheentupa J 1989 The neurohypophysis and water regulation. In: Brook P G D (ed) Clinical paediatric endocrinology, 2nd edn. Blackwell Scientific, Oxford, pp. 278–306

Paper 8 *QUESTIONS*

Question 8.1

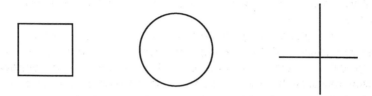

1. At what age would you expect a child to copy the above shapes correctly?

Question 8.2

These are the ECG traces from three healthy children with no cardiovascular problems.

A

B

C   V4R   V6

1. Which trace is from the youngest and which is from the oldest child?
2. If the bottom trace were found in a 4-month-old child with cyanotic heart disease, what would you suspect?

Question 8.3

These are the cardiac catheterization results from a 5-year-old boy:

	Oxygen saturation (%)	Blood pressure (mmHg) (systolic/diastolic)
Left ventricle	96	160/65
Left atrium	96	—
Thoracic aorta	96	80/60

1. What is the most likely diagnosis?
2. What abnormality may his ECG show?

Question 8.4

Shortly after vaccination a female infant became pale, limp and developed upper airways obstruction.

1. What is the diagnosis?
2. Name the drugs you would give to such a patient, including the dose and route of administration.

Question 8.5

An 11-month-old boy was investigated following recurrent subcutaneous abscess formation. The following results were obtained:

Haemoglobin	12 g/dl
White cell count	$14 \times 10^9/l$
Neutrophils	80%
ESR	Raised
Immunoglobulins	IgG, IgA and IgM elevated; IgE normal
Nitroblue tetraolium	Decreased reduction to insoluble blue formazan

1. What is the most likely diagnosis?

Question 8.6

A 10-year-old boy, following bedrest, developed a tender swollen calf followed by haemoptysis and chest pain. A family history of pulmonary emboli was obtained. Investigations revealed:

Haemoglobin	14 g/l
Platelet count	Normal
Partial thromboplastin time	Normal
Prothrombin time	Normal
Thrombin time	Normal
Bleeding time	4.5 min (normal up to 7 min)
Antithrombin-3	35%
Fibrinogen	3.2 g/l

1. What is the most likely cause of his chest pain?
2. What is the underlying cause of his illness?

Question 8.7

One parent has a sibling with cystic fibrosis and the other parent has no known family history of cystic fibrosis.

1. What is the risk their child will have cystic fibrosis?

Question 8.8

A 16-year-old boy with progressive darkening of the skin had the following results:

Blood film	Normal
Serum iron	Increased
Transferrin saturation	Increased
Total iron binding capacity	Decreased
Serum ferritin	Marked increase

One year later he developed polyuria and polydipsia. Urine testing was positive for glucose.

1. What is the most likely underlying diagnosis?
2. How would you confirm your diagnosis?

Question 8.9

A full-term male infant had an elevated TSH (280 mU/l) measured on his Guthrie test at 5 days of age. Results from subsequent investigations are:

Maternal thyroid function   Normal
Serum blood:
TSH   400 mU/l (normal <5 mU/l)
Free T4   <1.5 pmol/l (normal 8–26 pmol/l)
Free T3   1.5 pmol/l (normal 3–9 pmol/l)
123I scan   No radioiodine uptake

1. What is the most likely diagnosis?
2. His serum creatinine kinase was markedly elevated. What is the most likely explanation for this finding?

Question 8.10

A 10-month-old girl was investigated following a urinary tract infection. An ultrasound examination showed a dilated renal pelvis. A renogram was performed (Tc DTPA scan) — the background-subtracted scan is shown below; the lighter trace represents the left kidney and the darker line the right kidney. After 22 min frusemide (0.5 mg/kg) was given.

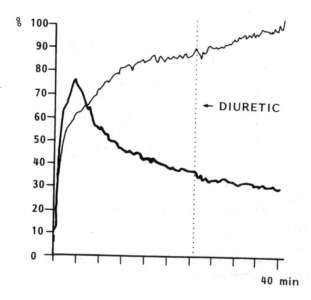

1. Comment on the renogram of the right kidney.
2. Comment on the renogram of the left kidney.

Paper 8 *ANSWERS*

Answer 8.1

1. $4\frac{1}{2}$ years (4–5 years is acceptable)

Discussion

When a child is able to use a pencil, copying drawings is a simple test of fine motor and 'conceptual development'. Examples of figures appropriate for different ages are:

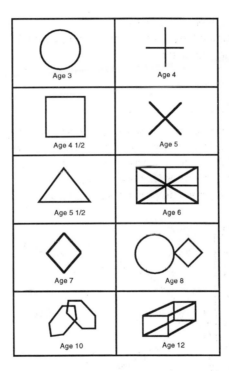

Answer 8.2

1. A = youngest
   C = oldest
2. Univentricular heart of left ventricular type with or without absent right atrioventricular connection

Discussion

Trace A is the neonatal ECG pattern, B the infant pattern, and C the adult pattern. The dominant R wave in V4R and dominant S wave in V6 is found in the first month of life. The dominant R wave in V6 and dominant R wave in V4R is found between 1 and 18 months. The adult pattern of dominant R wave in V6 and dominant S wave in V4R is found after this age. T-waves in V4R and V1 are upright at birth, but by 7 days should be inverted. The T-waves stay inverted in the majority of subjects until puberty when they become upright again.

The presence of an adult pattern (i.e. left ventricular dominance) in an infant with cyanotic heart disease suggests the possibility of a univentricular heart of left ventricular type with or without absent right atrioventricular connection. In the neonate, pulmonary atresia with intact ventricular septum or critical pulmonary stenosis with a small right ventricle should be considered.

Further reading
Shinebourne E A, Anderson R H 1985 Current paediatric cardiology. Oxford University Press, Oxford, pp. 49–56

Answer 8.3

1. Coarctation of the aorta
2. Left ventricular hypertrophy

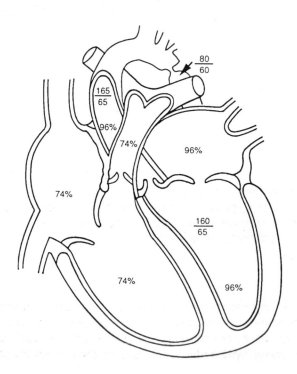

Discussion

The most likely diagnosis is coarctation of the aorta. Aortic stenosis may cause similar results but is far less common. Occasional patients may have both coarctation and aortic stenosis.

This asymptomatic boy had a post-ductal coarctation. His femoral pulses were smaller in volume than his right brachial pulse. There was no obvious radiofemoral delay. His right arm blood pressure revealed hypertension. Blood pressure should be measured in the right arm as the left subclavian artery may be involved in the coarctation. A mid-systolic ejection murmur was present at the upper left sternal border and a strong left ventricular pulse was felt.

Chest X-ray may be normal as cardiomegaly is infrequently seen on X-ray, even in older children, and ribnotching is seldom seen below the age of 5 years. Cross-sectional echocardiography did not reveal the coarctation.

Coarctation obstructs aortic blood flow and may depress left ventricular function. Left atrial and pulmonary venous and arterial pressures become raised. Systemic hypertension develops as a result of mechanical obstruction and increased renin production and fluid retention due to reduced renal perfusion.

Older children with coarctation are also at risk of infective endocarditis, aortic dissection and cerebrovascular accident. Operative repair or balloon dilatation angioplasty is indicated.

Left ventricular hypertrophy is commonly seen on the ECG of older patients with coarctation of the aorta. However, a normal ECG does not rule out the diagnosis of coarctation.

Further reading

Campbell A G M, McIntosh N (eds) 1992 Forfar and Arneil's Textbook of paediatrics, 4th edn. Churchill Livingstone, Edinburgh, pp. 683–685

Answer 8.4

1. Anaphylactic response to vaccine
2. 1 in 1000 adrenaline by deep intramuscular injection in a dose of 0.05 ml
   Chlorpheniramine maleate (Piriton) 2.5–5.0 mg intravenously   2 o o Mg/Kg
   Hydrocortisone (100 mg) intravenously   2 5 mg
   Oxygen by face mask

Discussion

Children who have been vaccinated should remain under observation until they are seen to recover from the procedure; it is not possible to specify an exact length of time. Anaphylactic reactions are rare but can be fatal. It is important to note that infants rarely faint and sudden loss of consciousness should be presumed to be an anaphylactic reaction in the absence of strong central pulse (i.e. carotid), which persists during a faint or convulsion.

The following symptoms may be observed during anaphylactic reaction:

— limpness and apnoea;
— upper airways obstruction; hoarseness and stridor as a result of angio-oedema involving the hypopharynx; epiglottis and larynx;
— lower airways obstruction;
— sinus tachycardia; profound hypotension in association with tachycardia; severe bradycardia;
— characteristic rapid development of urticarial lesions.

Adrenaline and appropriate sized oral airways must be available immediately whenever an immunization is given. Ideally the patient should be lying flat in the left lateral position, and if unconscious an oral airway inserted. Adrenaline is given by deep intramuscular injection unless there is a strong central pulse and the patient's condition is good. Oxygen should be given by a face mask and assistance sought. If appropriate, cardiopulmonary resuscitation should be performed. Piriton and hydrocortisone may be given to prevent further deterioration in severely affected cases. If there is no improvement in the patient's condition in 10 min, the dose of adrenaline may be repeated up to a maximum of three doses. All cases should be admitted to hospital for observation, and the reaction reported to the Committee of Safety of Medicines.

Further reading
Department of Health 1992 Immunisation against infectious disease. HMSO, London, pp. 9–10   (See 1996 Ed. pp. 41–42)

Answer 8.5

1. Chronic granulomatous disease

Discussion
Chronic granulomatous diseases are a group of disorders of the oxidative metabolism of phagocytes resulting in impairment of intracellular killing of catalase-positive bacteria, fungi or other microbes. *Staphylococcus aureus* is the most common infecting agent. Catalase-positive, Gram negative bacteria including *Escherichia coli*, Klebsiella and entero bacteria species, *Seratia marcescens*, salmonella and pseudomonas species account for approximately 30% of infections. Fungal pathogens also represent frequent and important causes of infection.

The nature of clinical infections in chronic granulomatous disease largely reflects an inability of circulating phagocytes to kill invading bacteria or fungi at sites of heavy colonization on or beneath skin or mucous membranes.

Inflammatory lesions of the skin or subcutaneous tissues, perianal abscesses, ulcerative stomatitis, conjunctivitis and pneumonitis are common clinical features.

The demonstration of impaired intracellular bactericidal activity by neutrophils, eosinophils or mononuclear phagocytes remains a definitive diagnostic test for chronic granulomatous disease. However, the nitroblue tetrazolium dye test may be used as a screening procedure. Oxidized nitroblue tetrazolium is colourless, but when reduced by superoxide, it precipitates in the cytosol as blue formazan. The reduced rate of conversion of oxygen to hydrogen peroxide can be quantitated by the nitroblue tetrazolium test.

Laboratory findings of leucocytosis, elevated ESR, and high IgG, IgA and IgM are also suggestive of chronic granulomatous disease. Biopsy tissue almost always reveals granulomas at sites of infection.

Further reading
Mouy R, Fischer A, Vilmer E, Seger R, Griscelli C 1989 Incidence, severity and prevention of infection in chronic granulomatous disease. Journal of Pediatrics 114: 555–560

Answer 8.6

1. Pulmonary embolus
2. Congenital antithrombin-3 deficiency

Discussion
The most likely cause of his chest pain is a pulmonary embolus secondary to a deep vein thrombosis. Antithrombin-3 is the main physiological inhibitor of coagulation. It is also an essential cofactor for heparin therapy. Thus deficiency may produce heparin resistance. The homozygous state is probably incompatible with life. Heterozygotes have a thrombotic tendency. Oral anticoagulant therapy and specific replacement concentrates can control the disorder. Acquired antithrombin-3 deficiency may occur in liver disease, nephrotic syndrome and protein calorie malnutrition.

Further reading
Campbell A G M, McIntosh N (eds) 1992 Forfar and Arneil's Textbook of paediatrics, 4th edn. Churchill Livingstone, Edinburgh, p. 953

Answer 8.7

1. 1 in 150 for each pregnancy

Discussion

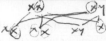

Risks are calculated by multiplying the chance that each parent is a carrier of the cystic fibrosis gene. In this example, the answer is obtained by multiplying $\frac{2}{3}$ (the chance the sibling is a carrier) and $\frac{1}{25}$ (the general carrier rate, which is the risk that the spouse is a carrier) and $\frac{1}{4}$ (the odds per pregnancy of producing a child with cystic fibrosis if both parents are carriers).

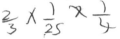

$$\frac{2}{3} \times \frac{1}{25} \times \frac{1}{4}$$

	Risk for each pregnancy
Both parents are carriers	1 in 4
One parent is a sibling of an individual with CF; the other is a known carrier	1 in 6
Both parents are siblings of individuals with CF	1 in 9
One parent has CF; the other parent has no known family history of CF	1 in 50
One parent is a known carrier of the CF gene; the other has no known family history of CF	1 in 100
One parent is a sibling of an individual with CF; the other has no known family history of CF	1 in 150
One parent is an aunt or uncle of an individual with CF; the other has no known history of CF	1 in 150/1 in 200
Both parents have no known family history of CF	1 in 2500

Further reading

Phelan P D, Landau L I, Olinsky A 1990 Respiratory illness in children. Blackwell Scientific, Oxford, pp. 192–193

Answer 8.8

1. Haemochromatosis
2. Liver biopsy

Discussion

This boy has haemochromatosis, due to an inborn error of metabolism resulting in excessive iron absorption from the gastrointestinal tract. He has developed diabetes.

Liver biopsy in patients with haemochromatosis shows marked iron deposition in liver cells and in Kupffer reticuloendothelial cells. Similar liver histology is found in children with thalassaemia and iron overload secondary to repeated transfusions. However, the blood film in such children would show hypochromia and microcytosis. There is a rare congenital sideroblastic anaemia, often X-linked, which presents in childhood with anaemia and splenomegaly and ultimately may lead to endocrine, liver and cardiac damage through iron overload. The sideroblastic anaemias are characterized by a dimorphic blood film. In patients with haemochromatosis, diabetes can result from pancreatic damage caused by excessive iron deposition ('bronzed diabetes'). Cardiomyopathy is another complication. In children with haematological causes of iron overload, desferrioxamine has been used to reduce the iron overload. Venesection therapy has improved survival in primary haemosiderosis.

Further reading

Campbell A G M, McIntosh N (eds) 1992 Forfar and Arneil's Textbook of paediatrics, 4th edn. Churchill Livingstone, Edinburgh, pp. 1214

Answer 8.9

1. Congenital hypothyroidism
2. Primary hypothyroidism, which may cause a false positive creatinine kinase test

Discussion

The TSH level measured in the serum and on the Guthrie test were markedly elevated. Free T4 and T3 are at the lower end of the normal range. [123]I scan showed no evidence of thyroid tissue. These results are consistent with a diagnosis of congenital hypothryoidism.

Congenital hypothyroidism has an overall prevalence of 1 in 4000 live births. Ninety-five per cent of all cases are sporadic, and 5% are genetic, usually reflecting a dyshormogenesis. There is a 2:1 female:male predominance.

Most cases of congenital hypothyroidism are detected by newborn screening tests which must always be confirmed by thyroid function tests on a venous blood sample. Certain clinical features of hypothyroidism may lead to suspicion of the diagnosis before screening tests are available. The signs and symptoms of congenital hypothyroidism are:

Large fontanelles	Prolonged jaundice
Umbilical hernia	Constipation
Macroglossia	Lethargy
Mottled, dry skin	Difficult feeding
Hypotonia	Cool skin
Abdominal distension	Sleeps through the night (newborn
Oedema	period)
Hoarse cry	Hypothermia
Respiratory distress	Goitre (rare)

In addition, features that suggest the possibility of hypopituitarism such as hypoglycaemia, micropenis and midline defects, should lead to evaluation for secondary hypothyroidism. Goitres are rarely present in these patients, even when dyshormogenesis is the cause. Goitres, however, may occur in the case of placental transmission of a goitrogen, and can be large enough to produce upper airways obstruction.

Treatment of congenital hypothryroidism involves replacement of thyroid hormone. With prompt and adequate treatment, children have potential for normal intellectual growth and development. Patients in whom treatment is begun before 6 weeks of age have an average IQ of 100. If treatment is begun at 6 weeks–3 months, the average IQ decreases to 95; at 3–6 months, 75; after 6 months, 55 or less. If an infant has evidence of congenital hypothyroidism on the basis of the newborn screening tests, but a firm diagnosis cannot be made speedily, treatment with thyroxine should be commenced.

The results of the serum creatinine kinase must be interpreted with caution. Primary hypothyroidism may cause a false positive creatinine kinase test. Causes of raised plasma creatinine kinase include:

— artefactual: due to in vitro haemolysis, using most methods;
— physiological: neonatal period (slightly raised) during and for a few days after parturition;
— marked increase: shock and circulatory failure, myocardial infarction, muscular dystrophies and rhabdomyolysis;
— moderate increase: muscle injury, after surgery (for about 1 week);
— physical exertion: there may be a significant rise in plasma activity after only moderate exercise, muscle cramp following an epileptic fit, or after intramuscular injection;
— hypothyroidism (thyroxine may influence the catabolism of the enzyme);
— alcoholism (possibly partly due to alcoholic myositis);
— some cases of cerebrovascular accident and head injury.

Plasma creatinine kinase activity is raised in all types of muscular dystrophy such as Duchenne's, but not usually in neurogenic muscle disease such as poliomyelitis, myasthenia gravis, multiple sclerosis or in adults with Parkinson's disease.

Further reading

Barnes N D 1985 Screening for congenital hypothyroidism: the first decade. *Archives of Disease in Children* 60: 587–592
Campbell A G M, McIntosh N (eds) 1992 Forfar and Arneil's Textbook of paediatrics, 4th edn. Churchill Livingstone, Edinburgh, pp. 1117–1119

Answer 8.10

1. Normal drainage of the right kidney
2. Progressive uptake of isotope, with no response to frusemide. The child has an obstructed left ureter

Discussion

A DMSA scan is a static scan and assesses kidney size and scar formation. A DTPA scan assesses dynamic function and can be used to calculate glomerular filtration rate of each kidney.

Following a left pyeloplasty the renogram curve of the left kidney has returned to normal. Excretion occurred well before the diuretic was injected.

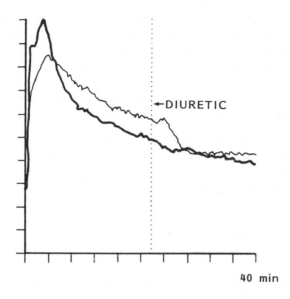

40 min

The renogram curve shows three classic phases. The first is a rapid rise in activity for a few seconds after the intravenous injection of isotope. This reflects the vascular supply to the kidney, and also the speed of injection. After a few seconds the rapid rise is replaced by a more gradual slope which reflects renal handling of isotope as it is taken up by the kidneys and passes down the nephrons. The curve rises because at this time more isotope is being extracted by the kidney than is leaving it by excretion. This second phase reaches a peak at 2–5 min, at which time about 5% of the injected dose is in each kidney. Following the peak, the curve descends as isotope excretion becomes greater than absorption. This coincides with the first appearance of activity within the bladder. This third phase is highly sensitive to abnormalities of the outflow tract and a normal curve excludes even trivial obstruction. If a kidney is non-functioning, the unsubtracted renogram curve will be identical to the blood background curve and the background subtracted curve will be flat.

At low flow rates the non-obstructed, dilated urinary tract will appear obstructed because of stasis of isotope. However, at high flow rates initiated by frusemide, the isotope will be washed out. The truly obstructed urinary tract will be obstructed at both low and high flow rates, as in this case.

The main indications for a renogram are:

— measurement of parenchymal function;
— suspected obstruction;
— evaluation of medical or surgical treatment;
— screening for renovascular hypertension when a renal artery stenosis delays the arrival and diminishes the amount of isotope reaching the parenchyma.

Further reading

Gordon I (ed) 1986 Diagnostic imaging in paediatrics. Chapman and Hall, London, pp. 135–136

Paper 9 *QUESTIONS*

Question 9.1

A 10-year-old girl presents with a 2-week history of being generally unwell followed by the onset of jaundice. There has been no foreign travel and no contact with anyone with jaundice. The parents were born in England, although all four grandparents are Mediterranean.

Blood tests:
Erythrocyte sedimentation rate   6 mm/h
Unconjugated bilirubin   75 μmol/l
Conjugated bilirubin   23 μmol/l
Gamma glutamyl transferase   124 IU/l
Alkaline aminotransferase   2771 IU/l
Alkaline phosphatase   428 IU/l
Albumin   48 g/l
Urinalysis:
Bilirubin   Positive
Urobilinogen   Negative
Stools   Normal colour

1. What is the most likely diagnosis?
2. Should the child be kept off school?

Question 9.2

A healthy boy is able to stand on one foot for a few seconds and can ride a tricycle. He is dry by night and able to discriminate colours.

1. At what age would a normal child be able to perform these tasks?
2. Using 1" square cubes, how high should he be able to build a tower?
3. Will he know what sex he is?

Question 9.3

Overleaf is part of the ECG trace from a 9-year-old girl who gave a history of recurrent episodes of 'feeling faint'.

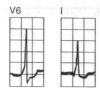

1. What two abnormalities does her ECG trace reveal?
2. What is the most likely diagnosis?

Question 9.4

These are the cardiac catheter findings of a 1-year-old boy who was found to have a heart murmur.

	Oxygen saturation (%)	Blood pressure (mmHg) (systolic/diastolic)
Right atrium	74	—/6
Right ventricle	86	45/6
Pulmonary artery	86	45/20
Left atrium	96	—/7
Left ventricle	97	100/70
Aorta	97	100/70

1. What is the diagnosis?
2. Will this child require antibiotic prophylaxis for dental procedures?

Question 9.5

A 4-year-old boy had a Mantoux test with 0.1 ml of purified protein derivative (100 U/ml) injected intradermally into the skin on the volar aspect of his forearm. The reaction was read at 48 h. Induration of 12 mm measured transversely to the long axis of the forearm was noted. His sister had a reaction also, but the induration was only 6 mm in diameter at 48 h, although vesiculation was present. Neither child had had a BCG.

1. What is the interpretation of the boy's reaction?
2. How do you interpret his sister's reaction?
3. Give three causes of a false negative reaction to the Mantoux test?

Question 9.6

A 5-year-old boy with microcephaly, absent thumbs and weight below the 3rd centile for his age was investigated because of increasing pallor. The following results were obtained:

Haemoglobin	8 g/dl
Haemoglobin F	Raised
Mean corpuscular volume	107 fl
White cell count	$2.2 \times 10^9/l$
Reticulocytes	<1%
Bone marrow aspirate	Hypocellular marrow with reduction in all cellular elements

1. What is the most likely diagnosis?
2. What other investigation may help with the diagnosis?

Question 9.7

A 2-year-old boy with bad eczema was investigated for recurrent infections of his ears and chest. The following results were obtained:

Haemoglobin	14.0 g/dl
White cell count	$10.0 \times 10^9/l$
Platelet count	$20 \times 10^9/l$
IgA	Twice normal
IgG	Twice normal
IgM	Half normal
Isohaemogglutinins	Absent

1. What is the most likely diagnosis?
2. What is the mode of inheritance?

Question 9.8

A 5-year-old boy presents with a history of loose, smelly stools 'on and off' over the past few years. He had his appendix out 1 year ago. Following surgery, a right iliac fossa mass had occurred under the scar.

Full blood count	Normal
Blood film	Normal
Urea and electrolytes	Normal
Liver function tests:	
Alkaline phosphatase	975 IU/l (normal 200–900 IU/l)
Bilirubin	Not icteric
Protein	57 g/l (normal 52–78 g/l)

Albumin	43 g/l (normal 35–45 g/l)
Alanine aminotransferase	47 IU/l (normal <40 IU/l)
Jejunal biopsy	Normal
Barium meal and follow through	Normal

1. What further investigation would most help towards making a diagnosis?
2. What is the cause of the iliac fossa mass?

Question 9.9

A 2-week-old male infant presents to hospital with a 1-week history of persistent vomitting and increasing lethargy. On examination the infant is 10% dehydrated and unwell. He has normal male external genitalia and both gonads are palpable. Blood results are:

Sodium	115 mmol/l
Potassium	7.2 mmol/l
Glucose	3.8 mmol/l

1. What is the most likely diagnosis?
2. What two investigations would be most helpful in confirming this diagnosis?

Question 9.10

A 3-year-old boy first presented at 3 months of age with bronchiolitis due to respiratory synctial virus but made a full recovery. At 18 months he required ventilation for pneumonia and at this time the blood results were:

Serum IgA	0.90 g/l (normal 0.15 – 0.88 g/l)
Serum IgG	0.29 g/l (normal 2.5 – 8.5 g/l)
Serum IgM	1.56 g/l (normal 0.43 –1.85 g/l)
Peripheral blood neutrophil count	0.05×10^9/l (normal $2.5 – 7.5 \times 10^9$/l)
Peripheral blood lymphocyte count	3.9×10^9/l (normal $1.5 – 4.0 \times 10^9$/l)
Neutrophil function tests	Normal

Height and weight at 3 years followed the 50th centile. A younger brother had meningococcal meningitis at the age of 15 months and a maternal uncle died unexpectedly in early childhood.

1. What is the most likely diagnosis?
2. Should he have any treatment now if he is well?

Paper 9 ANSWERS

Answer 9.1

1. Hepatitis A

Infectious mononucleosis, glandular fever or Epstein-Barr virus

Cytomegalovirus infection

2. No

Discussion

The commonest cause of infectious hepatitis in the UK is hepatitis A. If anti-hepatitis A IgM is not present, less common viral causes to look for are cytomegalovirus (more commonly causes a subclinical illness in young children) and Epstein-Barr virus (infectious mononucleosis). Hepatitis B and C are both spread by blood contact and are rare. The normal alkaline phosphatase is against an obstructive jaundice. The urinalysis cannot be explained by either an obstructive cause (typically pale stools and dark urine) or a haemolytic cause (normal stools and urine). The child's Mediterranean ancestry is a 'red herring'.

Bilirubin cannot be detected in normal urine as the plasma concentration of water-soluble conjugated bilirubin (<3.0 μmol/l) is too low to exceed the renal threshold. When conjugated bilirubin increases above 25 μmol/l in the plasma, it can be detected in the urine. Unconjugated bilirubin is not water soluble and therefore never appears in the urine from healthy kidneys irrespective of the plasma concentration (hence haemolytic anaemias are 'acholuric').

Urobilinogen is produced in the intestine by the action of bacteria on conjugated bilirubin excreted in the bile. Most of this is excreted in the faeces, contributing to the normal brown colour of the stools. However, a small amount is excreted by the kidneys into the urine (this makes up a negligible part of the colouring matter of the normal urine). This is increased in both haemolytic jaundice and in the pre-icteric and recovery phases of infective hepatitis.

The initial biochemical changes in infective hepatitis are due to mild hepatocellular damage — raised serum transaminases and an increased excretion of urobilinogen in the urine prior to the onset of jaundice. Once jaundice is established (clinically detectable when total plasma bilirubin >35 μmol/l), bilirubin appears in the urine without urobilinogen (because liver function is so poor that there is little bilirubin entering the small intestine) and the serum transferases become markedly increased. During recovery, bilirubin disappears from the urine and urobilinogen reappears.

Hepatitis A is most infectious in the period before onset of jaundice. However, it is a notifiable disease. The lack of an obvious contact is not unusual as:

— jaundice occurs in a minority of children, the majority experiencing only a gastrointestinal illness or being asymptomatic;
— the illness can be contracted from infected water or food;
— the incubation period can be as long as 6 weeks;
— the index case is likely to have been in the pre-icteric phase.

Further reading

Campbell A G M, McIntosh N (eds) 1992 Forfar and Arneil's Textbook of paediatrics, 4th edn. Churchill Livingstone, Edinburgh, pp. 545–551

Answer 9.2

1. 3 years old
2. 9"
3. Yes

Discussion

The following tables allow rapid assessment of developmental age. The boxes corresponding to the child's chronological age (horizontal axis) are filled in against the age-related developmental items on the left. One box must be filled in for each item achieved. Ninety per cent of children will complete items above the black line. Those 10% scoring below the line should be re-assessed within 1 month. Allowance must be made for prematurity when filling in these charts.

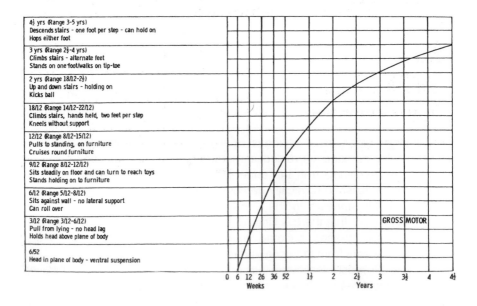

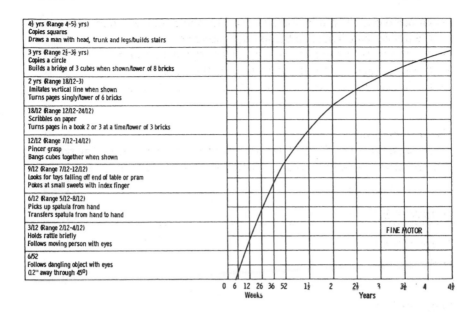

4½ yrs (Range 4-5½ yrs)
Copies squares
Draws a man with head, trunk and legs/builds stairs

3 yrs (Range 2½-3½ yrs)
Copies a circle
Builds a bridge of 3 cubes when shown/tower of 8 bricks

2 yrs (Range 18/12-3)
Imitates vertical line when shown
Turns pages singly/tower of 6 bricks

18/12 (Range 12/12-24/12)
Scribbles on paper
Turns pages in a book 2 or 3 at a time/tower of 3 bricks

12/12 (Range 7/12-14/12)
Pincer grasp
Bangs cubes together when shown

9/12 (Range 7/12-12/12)
Looks for toys falling off end of table or pram
Pokes at small sweets with index finger

6/12 (Range 5/12-8/12)
Picks up spatula from hand
Transfers spatula from hand to hand

3/12 (Range 2/12-4/12)
Holds rattle briefly
Follows moving person with eyes

6/52
Follows dangling object with eyes
(12" away through 45°)

FINE MOTOR

0 6 12 26 36 52   1½   2   2½   3   3½   4   4½
      Weeks   Years

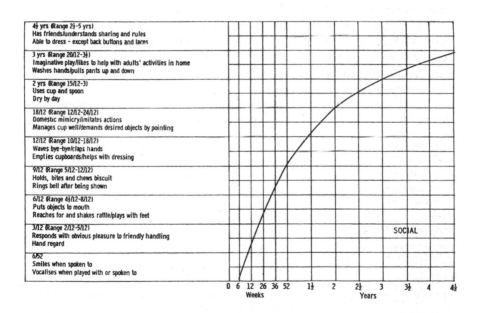

4½ yrs (Range 2½-5 yrs)
Has friends/understands sharing and rules
Able to dress - except back buttons and laces

3 yrs (Range 20/12-3½)
Imaginative play/likes to help with adults' activities in home
Washes hands/pulls pants up and down

2 yrs (Range 15/12-3)
Uses cup and spoon
Dry by day

18/12 (Range 12/12-24/12)
Domestic mimicry/imitates actions
Manages cup well/demands desired objects by pointing

12/12 (Range 10/12-18/12)
Waves bye-bye/claps hands
Empties cupboards/helps with dressing

9/12 (Range 5/12-12/12)
Holds, bites and chews biscuit
Rings bell after being shown

6/12 (Range 4½/12-8/12)
Puts objects to mouth
Reaches for and shakes rattle/plays with feet

3/12 (Range 2/12-5/12)
Responds with obvious pleasure to friendly handling
Hand regard

6/52
Smiles when spoken to
Vocalises when played with or spoken to

SOCIAL

0 6 12 26 36 52   1½   2   2½   3   3½   4   4½
      Weeks   Years

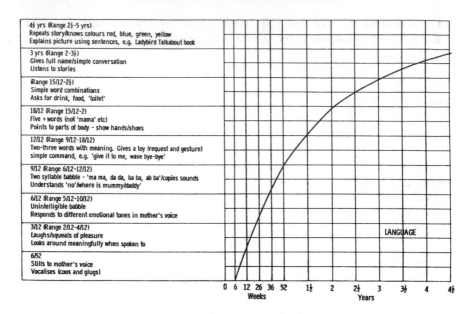

4½ yrs (Range 2½-5 yrs)
Repeats story/knows colours red, blue, green, yellow
Explains picture using sentences, e.g. Ladybird Talkabout book

3 yrs (Range 2-3½)
Gives full name/simple conversation
Listens to stories

(Range 15/12-2½)
Simple word combinations
Asks for drink, food, 'toilet'

18/12 (Range 15/12-2)
Five + words (not 'mama' etc)
Points to parts of body – show hands/shoes

12/12 (Range 9/12-18/12)
Two-three words with meaning. Gives a toy (request and gesture)
simple command, e.g. 'give it to me, wave bye-bye'

9/12 (Range 6/12-12/12)
Two syllable babble – 'ma ma, da da, ba ba, ab ba'/copies sounds
Understands 'no'/where is mummy/daddy'

6/12 (Range 5/12-10/12)
Unintelligible babble
Responds to different emotional tones in mother's voice

3/12 (Range 2/12-4/12)
Laughs/squeals of pleasure
Looks around meaningfully when spoken to

6/52
Stills to mother's voice
Vocalises (coos and glugs)

LANGUAGE

0 6 12 26 36 52   1½   2   2½ 3   3½   4   4½
Weeks   Years

Answer 9.3

1. Short P–R interval
ECG delta wave on the QRS complex
2. Wolff–Parkinson–White syndrome

Discussion

This child was suffering from recurrent attacks of supraventricular tachycardia due to Wolff–Parkinson–White syndrome. The ECG changes in this syndrome include:

— a short P–R interval
— initial slurring of the QRS complex
— prolonged QRS duration

Wolff–Parkinson–White syndrome is due to an anomalous conduction pathway (bundle of Kent) between the atrium and ventricle by-passing the AV node. The atrial impulse travels down the normal and anomalous pathways at the same time, but conduction is faster down the latter. Thus, the anomalous impulse reaches the ventricles earlier than the normally conducted impulse and results in the early delta wave of the QRS complex and hence a short P–R interval. Further transmission is slow into the ventricular muscle and the impulse conducted through the AV node overtakes and records the rest of the QRS complex.

This child developed recurrent episodes of reciprocating tachycardia due to block of conduction from the atria to ventricles (anterogradely) via the bundle of Kent. The impulse passes normally through the AV node only. However, this impulse is able to pass back through the bundle of Kent to the atria and back via the AV node again. This creates a circus movement between the normal pathway of conduction and the bundle of Kent producing a tachycardia.

Further reading

Park M K, Guntheroff W G 1992 How to read pediatric ECGs, 2nd edn. Mosby Yearbook, St. Louis

Answer 9.4

1. Ventricular septal defect
2. Yes

Discussion

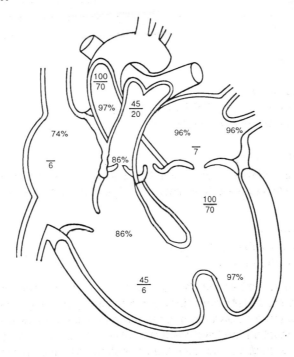

The murmur of a ventricular septal defect is often not heard in the first few days of life. Manifestations of the left-to-right shunt are not present at birth and may not appear until late infancy. Pulmonary vascular resistance is elevated in the fetus and the newborn. It usually falls over the first week of life, but may remain high for several months.

The haemodynamic consequences of a ventricular septal defect depend on the size of the left-to-right shunt, which is a function of the actual size of the defect itself and the relative pulmonary and systemic resistance. Left-to-right shunting at the ventricular level results in increased pulmonary blood flow and volume overload of the left ventricle. The increased volume work by the left ventricle is accomplished at the expense of an increased end diastolic filling pressure, which is reflected in increased left atrial and, ultimately, increased pulmonary venous pressure. A combination of increased blood flow and elevated pulmonary venous pressure produces increased hydrostatic pressure within the pulmonary capillary bed, which may result in accumulation of pulmonary interstitial fluid. Decreased pulmonary compliance with increased work of breathing accounts for early manifestations of congestive cardiac failure. More severe failure causing alveolar fluid collection can interfere with pulmonary gas exchange as well. One of the major concerns of a large ventricular septal defect is that pulmonary vascular obstructive disease may develop as early as 2 years of age and may result in the development of Eisenmenger's syndrome.

All patients with a ventricular septal defect, regardless of its size, are at risk of development of bacterial endocarditis. Standard recommendations for antibiotic prophylaxis should be encouraged for these patients unless spontaneous closure occurs. Surgical repair reduces risk, but does not completely eliminate it, especially if there is a residual defect.

Answer 9.5

1. Positive Mantoux test
2. Positive Mantoux test
3. Faulty injection (i.e. subcutaneous injection)
   Severe illness
   Measles
   Malnutrition
   Hodgkin's disease
   Sarcoidosis
   Miliary tuberculosis

Discussion

Induration of >10 mm is interpreted as positive for past or present infection with mycobacterium tuberculosis. If vesiculation is present, regardless of the amount of induration, this is also regarded as a positive reaction.

The tuberculin test has been the traditional method of diagnosing tuberculosis infection and the intradermal (Mantoux) using the equivalent of 5 IU of Tween-stabilized purified protein derivative (PPD) tuberculin is the test of choice in clinical practice. An intradermal injection of 0.1 ml of PPD tuberculin is given into the skin of the volar aspect of the forearm. A discreet pale wheal of 5 –10 mm should be produced when the exact amount of fluid (0.1 ml) is injected intradermally. The reaction is read 48–72 h after injection and is recorded as the diameter of induration in mm measured transversally to the long axis of the forearm. Erythema without induration is often difficult to interpret, but is not generally considered evidence of tuberculosis infection. If there is doubt then the test should be repeated because a subcutaneous injection can give erythema without induration.

Further reading
Strake J R 1988 Modern approach to the diagnosis and treatment of tuberculosis in children. Pediatric Clinics of North America 35: 441–464

Answer 9.6

1. Fanconi's anaemia
2. Examination of bone marrow chromosomes

Discussion
Fanconi's anaemia (congenital bone marrow aplasia) is inherited in an autosomal recessive fashion with a heterozygote frequency of 1 in 300 people. Half have typical physical findings which may include: hyperpigmentation, café-au-lait spots, microsomy, thumb anomalies, hypergenitalia, renal anomalies, ear anomalies, skeletal anomalies, micro-ophthalmia and mental retardation.

Haematological changes may not be apparent for several years. Initially patients may develop thrombocytopenia followed by a progressively increasing pancytopenia. HbF levels are often increased. Examination of bone marrow chromosomes is the investigation of choice in this child. It will show various spontaneous and induced chromosomal defects, including chromatid and chromosome breaks, constrictions and translocations. Fanconi's anaemia is one of the DNA repair disorders and the features of the disease are presumably related to this. The mechanism, however, is not entirely clear.

Successful treatment may be accomplished with marrow transplantation. If not, death from haemorrhage or infection often occurs during the second decade.

Further reading
Alter B P et al 1978 Classification and aetiology of aplastic anaemias. Clinical Haematology 7: 431–466

Answer 9.7

1. Wiskott–Aldrich syndrome
2. X-linked disorder

Discussion

Wiskott–Aldrich syndrome includes recurrent infections, haemorrhage secondary to thrombocytopenia and eczema of the skin. Children often come to medical attention with otitis media or pneumonia caused by *Streptococcus pneumoniae* or *Haemophilus influenzae*. Septicaemia or meningitis may develop. Candida, cytomegalovirus and *Pneumocystis carinii* may also be responsible for significant infections. Disseminated herpes and lethal chickenpox have been reported.

Wiskott–Aldrich patients fail to produce antibodies to polysaccharides, leading to low or absent isohaemagglutinins. They do not produce antibody to capsular polysaccharides of pneumococci or *Haemophilus influenza*, which explains the patient's susceptibility to infection with encapsulated organisms.

Platelets are reduced in number ($15–30 \times 10^9/l$) and are very small. In addition to eczema, autoimmune diseases such as haemolytic anaemia, vasculitis and juvenile rheumatoid arthritis, may occur. A high incidence of malignancy, especially non-Hodgkin's lymphoma, is seen.

An HLA-matched bone marrow transplant from a matched sibling donor has a high rate of success. Patients without a donor may benefit from splenectomy which raises platelet levels in over 90% of cases.

Further reading

Campbell A G M, McIntosh N (eds) 1992 Forfar and Arneil's Textbook of paediatrics, 4th edn. Churchill Livingstone, Edinburgh, pp. 1315–1316

Answer 9.8

1. Sweat test
2. Meconium ileus equivalent

   Crohn's disease

Discussion

A sweat test is essential to confirm or exclude cystic fibrosis. The normal jejunal biopsy and contrast study exclude many of the small bowel causes of malabsorption and steatorrhoea but an exocrine cause remains a possibility. The mild biochemical derangement of liver function is not unusual in cystic fibrosis. Exact thresholds vary with different laboratories but a sweat sodium or chloride >80 mmol/l is diagnostic. The sample, which is obtained with the aid of pilocarpine iontophoresis to stimulate the sweat glands, should contain >100 mg of sweat. The test is usually unsuccessful before 6 weeks of age.

The child has no gastrointestinal symptoms but if these developed oral *N*-acetyl cysteine or gastrograffin enema would be appropriate first-line therapy for meconium ileus equivalent. Crohn's disease is very rare in this age group and small bowel contrast radiology would have shown abnormalities if this were the correct diagnosis.

Answer 9.9

1. Congenital adrenal hyperplasia due to 21-hydroxylase deficiency

Salt-wasting adrenal hyperplasia

Congenital adrenal hyperplasia

Adrenal hypofunction

2. Plasma 17-hydroxyprogesterone assay

Plasma aldosterone assay

Urine steroid assay

Discussion

This child has a salt wasting congenital adrenal hyperplasia due to 21-hydroxylase deficiency. This specific diagnosis can be made from the history and data provided.

The combination of a low plasma sodium with a high plasma potassium should always make one think of lack of mineralocorticoid and therefore an adrenal disorder. The normal glucose and genitalia make it unlikely that this is part of a more widespread endocrinopathy such as panhypopituitarism (in which there is usually micropenis and hypoglycaemia). In adrenal disorders the other insulin antagonists (glucagon, growth hormone and catecholamines) are all maintained and therefore hypoglycaemia is not such a prominent feature.

Given that the infant is male and has normal genitalia, there are only two possible adrenal enzyme deficiencies associated with the phenotype: 21-hydroxylase deficiency — the commonest form of congenital adrenal hyperplasia, occurring in the homozygous state in 1 in 5000 infants in the UK, and the less common 11β-hydroxylase (associated with salt retention and hypertension). The commoner 21-hydroxylase form may either give rise to:

a) a simple virilizing form without salt wasting, in which case the karyotypic female has masculinized genitalia at birth, occasionally so markedly virilized that the infant is thought to be a normal male;

b) renal salt wasting also due to an additional defect in mineralocorticoid biosynthesis leading to aldosterone deficiency.

Lesser degrees of hyponatraemia may be seen in the newborn period with pyloric stenosis and urinary tract infection. The clue in this case is the high potassium which accompanies hyponatraemia due either to hypoadrenalism or chronic end-stage renal failure.

Measurement of cortisol alone is not useful for diagnosis. In all forms of congenital adrenal hyperplasia cortisol levels are either low or normal (the latter because in the affected but unstressed infant, cortisol levels may be normal as the enzyme deficiency is seldom complete). Likewise, plasma ACTH does not discriminate between the different types as this is elevated in all congenital adenal hyperplasia cases due to the adrenal hypofunction. The two most helpful investigations are plasma 17-hydroxyprogesterone levels and plasma aldosterone assay. 17-Hydroxyprogesterone is raised in the 21-hydroxylase and 11β-hydroxylase deficiencies and low when the block in steroid biosynthesis occurs earlier in the pathway. Aldosterone is low or normal in 21-hydroxylase deficiency (depending on whether it is simple virilizing or salt wasting) and aldosterone is always low in 11β-hydroxylase deficiency. Urine steroid assays have largely been superceded by plasma assays except for the rarer enzyme defects.

Further reading

Campbell A G M, McIntosh N (eds) 1992 Forfar and Arneil's Textbook of paediatrics, 4th edn. Churchill Livingstone, Edinburgh, pp. 1133–1141

Answer 9.10

1. X-linked immunodeficiency with increased IgM
Type I dysgammaglobulinaemia
'Hyper IgM syndrome'

X-linked agammaglobulinaemia
(congenital agammaglobulinaemia, Bruton's disease)

Selective immunoglobulin deficiency
Selective hypogammaglobulinaemia

2. Regular intravenous immunoglobulin infusions

Regular oral antibiotics
Regular oral prophylaxis

Discussion

These data show low IgA and IgG concentrations in a child who has had a severe pneumonia. Respiratory synctical virus infection is common in winter epidemics in the UK and this is not significant. There is also relative and absolute neutropenia. The family history suggests an X-linked inheritance as the mother's brother and both her sons appear to have been affected.

There are many causes of increased susceptibility to infection and the terminology and investigations can be confusing. The commonest categories are:

— hypogammaglobulinaemias;
— T cell deficiencies;
— severe combined immunodeficiency (reduced numbers of B and T lymphocytes and impaired antibody production);
— defective phagocytic function (chronic granulomatous disease, Chediak-Higashi syndrome, opsonization failure);
— complement deficiency states, particularly C3;
— secondary immunodeficiency (corticosteroids, cytotoxics, irradiation, lymphoproliferative disorders of malignancy, post-splenectomy);
— deficiencies of host physical defences (cystic fibrosis, Kartagener's syndrome).

Primary B cell deficiencies give rise to antibody defects resulting in recurrent, invasive infections with pyogenic bacteria (*Staphylococcus aureus, Streptococcus pneumoniae*, β-haemolytic streptococcus, *Neisseria meningitis, Haemophilus influenzae*). These organisms and the resulting infections (pharyngitis, sinusitis, otitis media, pneumonia, meningitis) are similar to those affecting immunocompetent children of a similar age group, but differ in their frequency and severity. They do respond to aggressive antimicrobial treatment. Because the cellular immune response of T cells is intact, patients respond normally to viral, fungal and mycobacterial infections. A similar clinical picture is seen in children with C3 complement deficiency because this component is required for chemotaxis, immune adherence and mast cell degranulation and such patients are therefore also prone to pyogenic infections. Defects of complement other than C3 are not usually associated with an excess of infections.

The major variants of antibody defect are:

— transient hypogammaglobulinaemia of infancy; there is delayed production of antibody so that as transplacental IgG titres fall, the child becomes prone to infection for a few months until spontaneous recovery occurs, usually within the first year of life;
— X-linked agammaglobulinaemia (congenital agammaglobulinaemia, Bruton's disease); IgA, IgG and IgM are all decreased in serum. Hypogammaglobulinaemia presenting before 2 years of life is most commonly the sex-linked variety. Mothers are carriers;
— X-linked immunodeficiency with increased IgM concentration; there is marked deficiency of serum IgA and IgG but normal or elevated IgM. Peripheral lymphocytes circulate in normal numbers but they are limited to production of IgM and sometimes IgD. There is often an associated haematological disorder (neutropenia, haemolytic anaemia or thrombocytopenia). There is autosomal dominant inheritance in 25% of cases, eosinophilia in 20%, and death from overwhelming infection in 10%;
— selective deficiencies; both IgG subclass and IgA deficiencies are recognized;
— acquired hypogammaglobulinaemia; the most common form of

immunodeficiency occurring in either sex at any age, usually without any known causative factor.

Provided diagnosis of hypogammaglobulinaemia is made before infection produces permanent damage (e.g. deafness secondary to meningitis or recurrent middle ear infections, bronchiectasis), the prognosis is greatly improved by regular intravenous administration of gammaglobulin, which is almost pure IgG, in doses adequate to maintain a serum concentration of IgG >2 g/l. This has superceded intramuscular injections which are painful. At age 3 years, this boy's serum IgG was 6.15 g/l (normal range 3.5–15 g/l) although serum IgA concentrations remained low. The half-life of circulating immunoglobulin dictates that the infusion be repeated every 2–6 weeks. Prophylaxis with gammaglobulin prevents invasive bacterial infections but, in a few instances, antibiotic prophylaxis is also necessary to control chronic sinusitis, most commonly due to *Haemophilus influenzae*.

Further reading

Milner A D, Hull D 1992 Hospital paediatrics, 2nd edn. Churchill Livingstone, Edinburgh, pp. 240–247
Rosen T S, Colten H R 1987 Primary immunodeficiencies and serum complement defects. In: Nathan D G, Oski F A (eds) Hematology of infancy and childhood, vol. 2, 3rd edn. W B Saunders, Philadelphia, pp. 878–899

Paper 10 *QUESTIONS*

Question 10.1

A 2-year-old child was suspected of having ketotic hypoglycaemia. The following results were obtained:

Lactate level	Normal
Insulin level	Decreased
Glucose level	Decreased
Cortisol	Increased
Growth hormone	Increased
β-hydroxybutyrate	Increased

1. Are the above results consistent with the suspected diagnosis?
2. If this child had ketotic hypoglycaemia, what would be the likely progosis?

Question 10.2

A 2-week-old boy was found to have a metabolic acidosis. High levels of leucine, isoleucine and valine were found in plasma and urine samples.

1. What is the diagnosis?

Question 10.3

The lecithin/sphingomyelin (L/S) ratio was determined in a group of 430 pregnant women. Following delivery, 356 neonates had no respiratory problems, although an L/S ratio of <2 had been recorded in 29 of them. 74 infants developed respiratory problems. Sixty-nine per cent of these had an L/S ratio of <2.

1. What is the sensitivity of this test?

Question 10.4

This is the ECG rhythm strip from a 6-year-old boy under observation on intensive care following cardiac surgery.

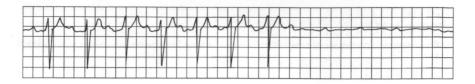

1. What two abnormalities are shown?

Question 10.5

A baby was born by an uncomplicated vaginal delivery at term and weighed 4.5 kg. At 12 h of age he was noticed to be cyanosed with a heart rate of 150 beats/min and a respiratory rate of 60 beats/min. ECG and chest X-ray were normal and the following blood gases were obtained from a right radial arterial cannula while the infant was breathing air:

pH	7.21
PaO_2	2.8 kPa
$PaCO_2$	4.0 kPa
Bicarbonate	12 mmol/l

A nitrogen washout test was then performed and after 10 min the following arterial blood sample was withdrawn from the same cannula:

pH	7.20
PaO_2	3.2 kPa
$PaCO_2$	4.1 kPa
Bicarbonate	13 mmol/l

1. What is the likely diagnosis?
2. What may be the most useful immediate treatment?

Question 10.6

A Schick test was performed on a teenage girl. This involved giving an interdermal injection of 0.1 ml Schick test toxin into the flexor surface of the left forearm, and 0.2 ml of Schick test control (inactivated toxin) into the corresponding position on the right forearm. Readings were made at 48 h and 7 days. No visible reaction was seen at these times on either arm.

1. What does the Schick test test for?
2. Is this patient immune?

Question 10.7

A baby born at 38 weeks gestation was noticed to be jaundiced on the 2nd day of life. The following results were obtained:

Haemoglobin	15 g/dl
Unconjugated bilirubin	280 µmol/l
Direct Coombs' test	Weakly positive
Blood group:	
Baby	Group A Rhesus positive
Mother	Group O Rhesus positive

1. What is the most likely diagnosis?

Question 10.8

A pregnant woman from South-East Asia is screened for hepatitis B and her blood tests showed:

HBsAg	Positive
HBeAg	Negative
Anti-HBe	Negative

Following a healthy pregnancy, a normal infant is born at term following a normal delivery.

1. What action, if any, should be taken following the delivery?

Question 10.9

This is the pedigree pattern for four generations of a family (shaded symbols represent affected individuals).

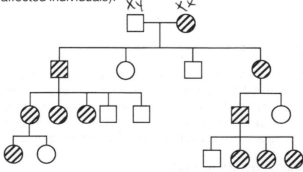

1. What kind of inheritance is shown?

Question 10.10

An 8-week-old boy was admitted with failure to thrive. The only abnormal finding on examination was hepatomegaly. Following a controlled fast, the following results were found:

Plasma glucose	1.6 mmol/l
Plasma cholesterol	5 mmol/l (normal 3.1–6.8 mmol/l)
Plasma triglycerides ↑	10.7 mmol/l (normal 0.6–1.7 mmol/l)
Plasma free fatty acids ↗	2.2 mmol/l (normal 0.3–1.5 mmol/l)
Plasma urate ↑	0.7 mmol/l (normal 0.12–0.42 mmol/l)
Plasma cortisol	760 nmol/l
Plasma gamma glutamyl ↗ transferase	253 U/l (normal up to 70 U/l)
Plasma alanine transferase ↑	263 U/l (normal up to 50 U/l)
Plasma alkaline phosphatase	180 U/l
Plasma bilirubin	5 mmol/l
Plasma albumin	35 g/l
Arterial blood gases:	
pH	7.38
PaCO$_2$	4 kPa
PaO$_2$	12 kPa
Bicarbonate	16 mmol/l
Base excess	6 mmol/l
Urinalysis	Positive for ketones

1. What is the most likely diagnosis?
2. Suggest three tests which would help confirm the diagnosis?

Paper 10 ANSWERS

Answer 10.1

1. Yes
2. Hypoglycaemia resolves with age

Discussion

Ketotic hypoglycaemia is a common disorder and most patients present between 18 and 24 months of age. Many are unable to fast for longer than 8–16 h before symptoms develop. Often there is a family history of transient hypoglycaemia and being small for gestational age in the neonatal period. As infants, they feed frequently and as toddlers are usually hungry on arising or after fasting for what would usually be a short time period for their age. They are not usually thin or obese.

Episodic hypoglycaemia occurs in situations where there is calorie deprivation. Examples include decreased intake during intercurrent illness, missing meals, or sleeping longer than usual. Acute hypoglycaemia is associated with the usual signs of lethargy, coma and seizures; it is thought to be due to decreased availability of glucose, impaired mobilization of muscle amino acids or poor gluconeogenesis. Due to 'accelerated starvation', free fatty acid oxidation leads to the markedly elevated plasma and urine ketone bodies, after which the disorder is named. The ability to fast improves with age, and most children outgrow this disorder by puberty. The disorder is inherited and tends to affect males more than females.

Treatment during acute episodes requires prompt correction of glucose, often with intravenous administration. Between episodes a high protein, high carbohydrate frequent feeding diet is given. Parents should be instructed in the measurement of urinary ketones and to increase glucose sources when ketones become positive or glucose intake decreases. Certain situations such as persistent vomiting or surgery will often require intravenous glucose to maintain normal glucose levels.

Further reading
Aynsley-Green A, Soltesz G 1985 Hypoglycaemia in infancy and childhood. Churchill Livingstone, Edinburgh

Answer 10.2

1. Maple syrup urine disease

Discussion

This boy has maple syrup urine disease which is caused by reduced activity of branched-chain oxoacid dehydrogenase. The incidence is 1 in 120 000 and inheritance is autosomal recessive. The characteristic smell of maple syrup may not present in the urine. The degree of severity varies depending on the residual activity of the enzyme involved. Severe acidosis, hypoglycaemia and hyperammonaemia may occur in the neonatal period, leading to seizures and death. Dialysis may be required. Mild cases may not be detected until late infancy when an intermittent illness results in decompensation with acidosis and lethargy.

Patients with appreciable residual enzyme activity may be treated with thiamine. Lack of response indicates a need for strict dietary control. This consists of a mixture of synthetic amino acids without the branched-chain amino acids leucine, isoleucine and valine. Small amounts of natural protein providing enough valine, leucine and isoleucine, are given to maintain normal blood levels.

Further reading

Zilva J F, Pannal P R, Mayne P D 1988 Clinical chemistry in diagnosis and treatment. Edward Arnold, London, p. 371

Answer 6.3

1. 69%

Discussion

The *sensitivity* of any test is a measure of its ability to distinguish as positive those patients who have the condition under investigation. The *specificity* is a measure of the ability to identify correctly those patients who do not have the condition. For example, suppose you took 'possession of functioning lungs' as a way of diagnosing asthma. You would identify correctly all patients with asthma, i.e. the sensitivity would be high, but since a substantial proportion of patients without functioning lungs will not have asthma, the specificity will be low.

$$\text{Sensitivity} = \frac{\text{number tested as positive}}{\text{total number with the condition}}$$

$$\text{Specificity} = \frac{\text{number tested as negative}}{\text{total number without the condition}}$$

Remember to calculate 69% of 74 to arrive at the number of infants with L/S ratios <2 who develop respiratory problems. The easiest way to work out the answer is to construct a table:

L/S ratio	No respiratory problems	Respiratory problems	Total
>2	327 (a)	23 (c)	350
<2	29 (b)	51 (d)	80
Total	356	74	430

$$\text{Sensitivity} = \frac{d}{c+d}$$

$$= \frac{51}{23+51} \times 100$$

$$= 69\%$$

Answer 10.4

1. First-degree heart block

Asystole

Discussion

First-degree heart block is produced by an abnormal delay in conduction through the AV node, resulting in prolongation of P–R interval beyond the upper limit of normal for the patient's age and heart rate. First-degree heart block is occasionally seen in healthy children. However, it may be associated with cardiac conditions such as: Ebstein's anomaly, atrial septal defect, rheumatic fever, myocardiopathies and digoxin toxicity.

Further reading

Park M K, Guntheroff W G 1992 How to read paediatric ECGs, 2nd edn. Mosby Yearbook, St. Louis

Answer 10.5

1. Transposition of the great arteries

Congenital cyanotic heart disease

2. Prostaglandin E infusion

Discussion

This is a term infant who is centrally cyanosed but with no clinical or radiological evidence to suggest respiratory disease apart from a mild tachypnoea. The most likely cause is, therefore, cyanotic congenital heart disease but this answer would score fewer marks as it is not a specific anatomical diagnosis. The commonest cause in the newborn period with normal ECG and chest X-ray is transposition of the great arteries and this is the best answer.

In this condition, the pulmonary and systemic circulations function in parallel and as soon as the foramen ovale and ductus arteriosus start to close, there is decreased mixing between the two circulations and systemic hypoxia and cyanosis develop. There is, therefore, often an initial 'honeymoon period' when the infant appears well. The tachypnoea is a result of hyperventilation in an effort to compensate for metabolic acidosis with respiratory alkalosis and indeed the arterial blood gas in air shows in addition to hypoxia, a low/normal $PaCO_2$ and a low pH. A chest X-ray may show the classic 'egg on side' appearance or pulmonary plethora, but these features are often seen with the benefit of hindsight and at the time of presentation the chest X-ray often appears normal. The importance of this is that it helps exclude a respiratory cause for the cyanosis. The ECG shows the normal pattern of right ventricular dominance seen in the immediate newborn period. There is no murmur.

The nitrogen washout test (also known as a hyperoxic test — an oxygen analyser should be used to demonstrate that the inspired oxygen concentration is continuously >90% for at least 10 min) has confirmed that no benefit will be gained by giving the infant oxygen. A prostaglandin E infusion should be started as some, but not all, infants will benefit from this as the prostaglandin maintains patency of the ductus arteriosus. If the arterial blood gases show an improvement in PaO_2 following this infusion, it should be continued until transfer to a cardiac centre where an urgent balloon septostomy is required to allow mixing of atrial blood. Although the infant is breathing normally and has no respiratory disease, he should be intubated and ventilated for transfer as a side-effect of prostaglandin infusion is apnoea. There is little to be gained by giving sodium bicarbonate to correct this mild degree of acidaemia and a further advantage of intermittent positive pressure ventilation is that the hypocapnia can be maintained, thus avoiding a profound acidosis. If the prostaglandin infusion is successful in improving the arterial oxygenation, the metabolic acidosis may improve and at least should not deteriorate further.

Following balloon septostomy and stabilization, the treatment of choice is corrective cardiac surgery in the first week of life involving a primary switch operation with connection of the main pulmonary artery to the right ventricle and anastomosis of the aorta and coronary arteries to the left ventricule.

Other causes of cyanotic congenital heart disease presenting in the first week of life are tricuspid atresia (with right-to-left shunt occurring at atrial level), total pulmonary atresia (with or without an intact ventricular septum), obstructive total anomalous pulmonary venous drainage (usually the infracardiac type) and Ebstein's anomaly (again with right-to-left shunt occurring at the atrial level). Atrioventricular canal defects, commonest in Down's syndrome babies, may present immediately in the newborn period or later depending on the degree of mixing of venous and arterial blood and hence cyanosis. Tetralogy of Fallot and non-obstructive total anomalous pulmonary venous drainage usually present after the first week of life.

Further reading
Milner A D, Hull D 1992 Hospital paediatrics, 2nd edn. Churchill Livingstone, Edinburgh, pp. 121–123

Answer 10.6

1. Determines whether a patient is immune to diptheria
2. Yes

Discussion

The Schick test is recommended for anyone who may be exposed to diptheria during the course of their work. In such cases immunity to diptheria should be ensured by means of a Schick test carried out at least 3 months after immunization is completed.

The following reactions may follow the Schick test:

a) Schick positive — an erythematous reaction occurs at the site of toxin injection, in 24–48 h persisting for several days. The control shows no reaction. In this case, the subject is not immune and needs to be immunized or reinforced;

b) negative and pseudo-reaction — both injection sites have similar reactions at 48–72 h. The reactions are due to hypersensitivity to the components of the test materials. The subject is immune and need not be immunized or reinforced;

c) positive and pseudo-reaction — both injection sites show reactions up to 48 –72 h but the reaction on the site the toxin was injected is larger and more intense. The control response fades considerably by the fifth day, leaving the positive effect clearly seen. Such combined reactors usually have a basal immunity to diphtheria and should not be immunized with a further full course of vaccine. Their immunity can successfully be reinforced by single injection of diptheria vaccine (low dose).

Further reading
Department of Health 1990 Immunisation against infectious disease. HMSO, London, pp 21–22

Answer 10.7

1. ABO haemolytic disease of the newborn

Discussion

In ABO haemolytic disease, jaundice usually presents in the first 24 h. The mother is usually blood group O and the baby either A or B. The Coombs' test is weakly positive and a large number of spherocytes in the blood film make the diagnosis likely. Demonstration of anti-A or anti-B IgG haemolysins in a maternal sample makes the diagnosis almost certain.

Although many mothers have incompatibility of their blood group with their fetus, haemolytic disease due to ABO incompatibility occurs only in approximately 1 in 150 of these deliveries. This is because most naturally occurring anti-A or anti-B in the mother is IgM and does not cross the placenta. Small quantities of anti-A or anti-B IgG are present but are usually bound rapidly by the fetus's tissue. Binding sites on fetal red cells are poorly developed.

Although ABO haemolytic disease causes up to two-thirds of cases of haemolytic disease of the newborn, it is seldom severe and jaundice usually needs little more than phototherapy for management. Exchange transfusion is rarely required.

Further reading

Campbell A G M, McIntosh N (eds) 1992 Forfar and Arneil's Textbook of paediatrics, 4th edn. Churchill Livingstone, Edinburgh, pp. 256–259

Answer 10.8

1. Immunization of infant against hepatitis B

Discussion

Hepatitis B virus infection may be transferred from mother to infant at any time during pregnancy or delivery and prevention of vertical transmission depends on the combination of passive and active immunization of infants at risk as soon as possible after birth. The prevalence of hepatitis B carriers varies widely in different populations of pregnant women and at present in the UK those screened for hepatitis B are women with recent acute hepatitis, ethnic groups other than caucasians of Northern or Western European origin, and caucasians with personal or family history, occupations or lifestyle suggestive of increased risk of exposure to hepatitis B infection (essentially those with known sexually transmitted diseases or who have abused drugs intravenously). This group will be screened initially for hepatitis B surface antigen and if this is present, further tests will delineate the degree of infectivity. If the mother is also positive for hepatitis e antigen, then she is highly infective. If the mother's blood contains anti-HBe antibodies, then her blood has a low infectivity. If the mother's blood is negative for both hepatitis B e antigen and the antibody, her blood is of intermediate infectivity.

Without immunization, 80% of infants of hepatitis B e antigen positive mothers will in the first few months of life develop hepatitis B carriage and a high risk of cirrhosis and hepatoma in later life. About 10% of infants of mothers who have anti-HBe antibodies will be infected. Only a small fraction of these develop acute hepatitis B. The risk to infants of carrier mothers who have neither hepatitis B e antigen or its antibody is intermediate between these and therefore still substantial.

At the time of birth, the baby should be delivered in an isolation room and cord blood taken to check the baby's hepatitis B status. Passive immunization should be given as soon as possible and certainly within 48 h, by deep intramuscular injection of human anti-hepatitis B immunoglobulin. The first dose of active hepatitis B immunization should be given at a different site at the same time and further doses of the vaccine given at 1 and 6 months.

At 1 year, all children who have been immunized against hepatitis B should be checked for hepatitis B antigens and antibody titres to check for adequate seroconversion. If the antibodies against hepatitis B surface antigen are not present in adequate concentration, a booster dose of hepatitis B vaccine is given at 1 year. It is also recommended that, at around the fifth birthday, a booster dose should be given to all children who have received hepatitis B vaccine at birth and responded.

Further reading

Department of Health 1992 Immunisation against infectious diseases. HMSO, London
Polakoff, Vandervelde 1980 Immunisation of neonates at high risk of hepatitis B in England and Wales. British Medical Journal 297: 249–253

Answer 10.9

1. X-linked dominant inheritance

Discussion

An X-linked dominant disorder is one in which the phenotypic features are manifest in both the heterozygous female and the hemizygous male. The pedigree resembles that of an autosomal dominant inheritance but in an X-linked disorder, an affected male transmits the disease to all his daughters and to none of his sons. In an autosomal dominant disorder, in contrast, an affected father should transmit the disease to half his daughters and half his sons equally. In an X-linked dominant disorder, affected females transmit the disease equally to sons and daughters, again half of whom on average will be affected. There are relatively few dominant disorders which are carried on the X-chromosome. The example shown is of vitamin D resistant rickets. In some X-linked dominant disorders the condition is lethal in utero for males and so only females appear to be affected (an example is incontinentia pigmenti).

This pedigree shows that the two affected males have each had three affected children but none of their sons has been affected. It cannot be said categorically that this is not the pedigree of an autosomal dominant disorder as there is a very small chance of only the father's daughters being affected. The question is what is the most likely inheritance pattern shown. The correct answer is X-linked dominant. If the candidate gave the answer as autosomal dominant, this would probably be accepted but would score much fewer marks than X-linked dominant.

Answer 10.10

1. Type I glycogen storage disease

   Glycogen storage disease
2. Liver biopsy

   Intravenous galactose test
   Glucagon test
   Oral glucose tolerance test

Discussion

Type I glycogen storage disease (also called Von Gierke's disease) is due to deficiency of the enzyme glucose-6-phosphatase. The presence of fasting hypoglycaemia with metabolic acidosis due to lactic acid, increased triglyceride and urate concentrations with hepatomegaly are highly suggestive of this diagnosis. In older children, clinical findings are usually a rounded 'doll's face', short stature, central obesity with marked hepatomegaly and hypotrophic muscles. The kidneys may also be enlarged. The child usually comes to attention because of recurrent hypoglycaemia with acidosis or failure to thrive.

Several inherited enzyme defects may interfere with the degradation of glycogen resulting in an increased glycogen content of various organs and an inability to release glucose as a fuel when exogenous supplies of glucose are limited. Glycogen is a polysaccharide in which glucose is stored in various organs but particularly the liver and the muscles. In liver, the major function of glycogen is to act as a reserve to provide glucose for export to other organs particularly the brain. In contrast, muscle glycogen functions as a local fuel during muscle contraction. The different enzyme defects which may interfere with glycogen degradation may therefore give rise to fasting hypoglycaemia if liver enzymes are involved or myopathy if muscle enzymes are involved.

In Type I glycogen storage disease, the deficiency of glucose-6-phosphatase results in a failure to dephosphorylate glucose-6-phosphate into glucose. This means that glucose production from both glycogenolysis and gluconeogenesis is blocked. However, glycogen can still be converted into pyruvate and this results in increased lactate production. Excess acetyl-CoA is also produced which is converted into fatty acids and cholesterol, explaining the hyperlipidaemia seen in this condition. Glucose-6-phosphate also accumulates but may be channelled via an alternative pathway into the production of urate leading to the hyperuricaemia which occurs in almost all patients eventually and may lead to nephropathy and gout.

The four helpful investigations are:

— an intravenous galactose test; intravenous infusion results in an elevation of blood lactate rather than glucose;
— a glucagon test; the administration of glucagon fails to increase the blood glucose concentration but results in a rise in lactic acid level;
— an oral glucose tolerance test; this is the safest of the three challenge tests and results in a decrease in blood lactate from an initially high fasting level to a near normal blood lactate level;
— an assay of glucose-6-phosphatase activity in a liver biopsy is the definitive diagnosis. Liver biopsy may also show some increase in the glycogen stored in the liver, as a percentage of wet weight, but this is not a requirement for diagnosis as the concentration of glycogen in the liver is influenced by various factors such as nutritional status, the timing of the biopsy in relation to meals and by hormonal stimuli. Accumulation of fat in the liver may be more striking than that of glycogen.

There is no curative treatment. Management is based on avoiding hypoglycaemic episodes in which case a normal intelligence should be the outcome. Daytime hypoglycaemia is avoided in a young infant by frequent (2 hourly) formula feeds. Overnight continuous nasogastric tube feeds are required. An alternative is to use a gastrostomy to allow continuous overnight feeding. As the child gets older, it is possible to introduce uncooked starch into the diet which has a slower gastric transit than glucose and allows a more gradual glucose release from the gut. The complications of hyperuricaemia can be avoided by treatment with allopurinol. Benign liver adenomas develop in a majority of patients in adult life.

The glucose-6-phosphatase enzyme system is complex and two other enzymes can give rise to a clinical picture very similar to that described above. For this reason, classic Von Gierke's disease is sometimes called glycogen storage disease Type 1A and the similar phenotypes due to defects of enzymes called translocases, which allow entry and exit of glucose-6-phosphate through the endoplasmic reticulum, are called Types 1B and 1C. Type 1B accounts for 15% of all cases of glucose-6-phosphatase deficiency and may be suspected from the associated neutropenia which is not a feature of Type 1A glycogen storage disease.

Paper 11 *QUESTIONS*

Question 11.1

This is the EEG from a 7-year-old girl.

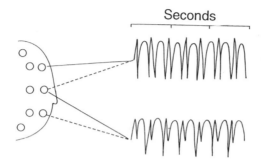

1. What does the EEG show?
2. What is the diagnosis?

Question 11.2

This ECG trace was taken from a neonatal patient.

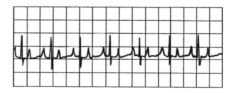

1. Give two abnormalities seen on this trace.

Question 11.3

A term infant develops cardiac failure in the first week of life. The infant is pink in air and pulses are collapsing but there is no cardiac murmur. Investigations show:

Electrocardiogram Normal
Chest radiograph Cardiomegaly
Echocardiogram Anatomically normal heart with normal connections
                and great vessels. The ductus arteriosus is closed

1. What is the diagnosis?
2. What other investigation would you suggest?

Question 11.4

The graph shows the percentage of normal adult immunoglobulins in fetal and post-natal life. C represents neonatal IgG.

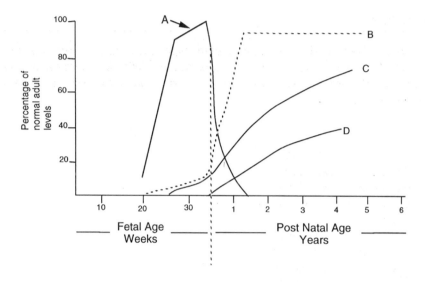

1. What do A, B and D represent?
2. Some transient diseases in the newborn may be caused by maternal IgG. Name five.

Question 11.5

A 14-year-old girl presents complaining of tiredness on most days during the last 6 months and frequent sore throats over that period. She is a vegan. Her periods started 2 years ago and she describes them as quite heavy. Investigations show:

Erythrocyte sedimentation ratio	7 mm/h
Haemoglobin	12.4 g/dl
Mean corpuscular volume	85 fl
Mean corpuscular haemoglobin	30 pg
White cell count	$7.1 \times 10^9/l$
Neutrophils	64.5%
Lymphocytes	27.7%
Monocytes	6.8%

Blood film	Normal
Paul Bunnell test	Negative
IgG to Epstein Barr viral capsid antigen	Present
IgG to Epstein Barr nuclear antigen	Not detected

1. What is the most likely diagnosis?

Question 11.6

A 3-week-old boy is admitted because of tachypnoea, vomiting, diarrhoea and irritability. He has a generalized afebrile seizure following admission and arterial blood taken immediately afterwards, while breathing room air, gives the following results:

pH	7.075
PaO_2	12.9 kPa
$PaCO_2$	2.33 kPa
Bicarbonate	5.1 mmol/l
Base excess	−23.6 mmol/l
Plasma:	
Sodium	137 mmol/l
Potassium	4.4 mmol/l
Urea	1.4 mmol/l
Creatinine	53 μmol/l
Glucose	1.5 mmol/l
Calcium	2.37 mmol/l
Albumin	37 g/l

1. What is the most likely explanation for these results?
2. Suggest three urine tests that would help define the exact diagnosis.

Question 11.7

A girl, the second of twins born at 27 weeks gestation, is found on routine screening at 6 days of age to have a thyroid stimulating hormone (TSH) concentration of 380 mU/l. The mother had taken no drugs during pregnancy and there is no family history of thyroid disease. She is started on 12.5 μg of thyroxine daily, increasing to 25 μg. At 6 months of age, her TSH is 50 mU/l with a total serum thyroxine of 131 mmol/l (normal range 53–135 mmol/l).

1. What is the most likely explanation for these results?

Question 11.8

A boy of 8 months presents with fever and on examination he has mild bruising and is hypotonic. Investigations give the following results:

Haemoglobin	9 g/dl
Platelet count	$300 \times 10^9/l$
White cell count	$16 \times 10^9/l$
Polymorphs	80%
Activated partial prothrombin time	120 s
Prothrombin ratio	8
Ammonia	195 mmol/l

1. What is the most likely diagnosis?
2. Give three causes to explain the ammonia level.

Question 11.9

A 13-year-old girl who has attended casualty has the following results:

	Arterial blood	Urine
pH	7.25	4.0
PaCO$_2$	4.0 kPa	
PaO$_2$	11.5 kPa	
Base excess	-12 mmol/l	
Bicarbonate	16 mmol/l	
Sodium	135 mmol/l	6 mmol/l
Osmolality	285 mOsmol/kg	550 mOsmol/kg
Glucose	13 mmol/l	
Prothrombin ratio	3.2	

4 h later the following results were obtained:

pH	7.35	7.5
PaCO$_2$	4.6 kPa	
PaO$_2$	11.0 kPa	
Base excess	-2 mmol/l	
Bicarbonate	25 mmol/l	
Sodium	135 mmol/l	100 mmol/l
Osmolality	280 mOsmol/kg	320 mOsmol/kg
Glucose	10.0 mmol/l	
Prothrombin ratio	3.2	

1. What is the most likely diagnosis based on the initial results?

2. From the data, what specific treatment has been given between the two
sets of results?

Question 11.10

An 18-month-old baby presented with fever and neck stiffness. Blood pressure
was 100/60 mmHg and heart rate 95 beats/min. Lumbar puncture gave the
following results:

White cell count	16×10^9/l
Polymorphs	80%
Red cell count	0/l
Protein	0.8 g/l
Glucose	0.6 mmol/l

The next day the baby had a generalized convulsion and the following results
were obtained

Plasma sodium	120 mmol/l
Plasma potassium	4.0 mmol/l
Plasma urea	3.0 mmol/l
Plasma calcium	2.4 mmol/l
Plasma albumin	35 g/l
Plasma glucose	4.2 mmol/l
Plasma osmolality	250 mOsmol/kg
Urine osmolality	320 mOsmol/kg

1. What biochemical diagnosis is appropriate?
2. How would you manage the fluid balance?

Paper 11 *ANSWERS*

Answer 11.1

1. Symmetrical 3/second spike/wave complexes
2. Primary generalized epilepsy of petit mal type (known as generalized minor motor seizure)

Discussion

The main clinical feature of a true petit mal attack is a sudden, brief (5–15 s and rarely longer than 30s), blank stare accompanied by unawareness and sometimes by flickering of the eyelids. There is usually amnesia of the event. Onset is usually between the ages of 5 and 15 years and it occurs more commonly in girls.

The EEG shows typical 3/s regular spike wave discharges. It is usually possible to be fairly certain about the diagnosis of petit mal absences from the history, and the true EEG generally confirms this. It is very rare for true petit mal epilepsy to be due to structural brain lesions and unusual for mental retardation or neurological deficit to be associated with it.

Prognosis is usually excellent with attacks often ceasing spontaneously after a few years. Features suggesting an excellent prognosis are: onset before the age of 10 years, a good initial response to drugs, lack of other types of seizure, normal mental and neurological status, and a typical EEG pattern.

Drug treatment is usually very effective and ethosuximide or sodium valproate are used.

Further reading

Brett E 1991 Paediatric neurology, 2nd edn. Churchill Livingstone, Edinburgh, pp. 346–359

Answer 11.2

1. 2:1 second-degree atrioventricular heart block
   Right atrial hypertrophy

Discussion

The heart rate is 120 beats/min which is normal for age. The rhythm is also regular. However, there are two P-waves before each R-wave. Only one of these P-waves is conducted with a regular P–R interval, that is second-degree atrioventricular block. Right atrial hypertrophy is suggested by a 3 mm P-wave.

Answer 11.3

1. Systemic arteriovenous malformation
2. Selective angiography

Discussion

The infant has cardiac failure but a normal heart. The increased cardiac output is necessary to maintain systolic blood pressure in the face of a low resistance left-to-right extracardiac shunt in the systemic circulation. The presence of collapsing pulses is the clue to the arterial run-off in diastole and although this is commonest in a patent ductus arteriosus, there are other causes (e.g. systemic arteriovenous malformation, aortic regurgitation).

A cranial or hepatic bruit, or the presence of a skin haemangioma (which can be associated with a consumptive thrombocytopenia – Kasabach–Merritt syndrome) may suggest the site of the arteriovenous malformation. In the absence of any clinical clue as to the site, selective angiography will be required. Pulmonary arteriovenous malformations also occur (which may be multiple and associated with facial telangectasia – Osler–Weber–Rendu syndrome) but cause cyanosis (the pressure in the pulmonary arteries exceeds that in the pulmonary veins and there is effectively right-to-left extracardiac shunt).

Answer 11.4

1. A = maternal IgG
   B = neonatal IgM
   D = neonatal IgA
2. Thyrotoxicosis
   Thrombocytopenia
   Lupus erythomatosus
   Myasthenia gravis
   Rhesus incompatibility

Discussion

Of the immunoglobulins, only IgG subclasses cross the placenta. Placental Fc receptors transport IgG subclasses and antibody actively, but somewhat selectively, across the placenta. In term infants, the infant:maternal ratio of total IgG is 1.8 but some IgG subclasses may have ratios of 1. Antibody crosses the placenta in a similar but variable manner. For example, the IgG infant:maternal ratio for tetanus toxoid is 1.9 and for IgG haemophilis polysaccharide antibody is 2.2.

Immunoglobulin decreases after birth, the nadir being 1 month after for IgG-3 and about 4 months for the other subclasses. Premature infants do not receive as much transplacental immunoglobulin as those born at term. Several studies involving administration of prophylactic gammaglobulin to very preterm infants have shown some reduction in infection but the advantages do not seem to be as great as might have been expected. IgG-1 and IgG-3 responses mature more rapidly than IgG-2 and IgG-4. Responsiveness to carbohydrate or polysaccharide antigens is usually impaired until 2 years of age. Total IgG reaches adult proportions by 5–7 years, IgG-2 and IgG-4 by 10–12 years, IgM by 1–2 years and IgA by 8–10 years.

Further reading

Watson J G, Bird A G 1989 Handbook of immunological investigation in children. John Wright, Bristol, pp. 214–240

Answer 11.6 11.5

1. Glandular fever

Discussion

Although this teenager is a vegan and has heavy periods, her red cell results are all within the normal range. These vary from laboratory to laboratory, but are approximately:

Haemoglobin	11.5–16.5 g/dl
Mean corpuscular volume	76–99 fl
Mean corpuscular haemoglobin	27–32 pg

Antibody present against Epstein-Barr viral capsid antigen but not the nuclear antigen is evidence of a fairly recent infection. However, as the ESR is low, the white cell count is not increased, the blood film does not show any atypical lymphocytes, and the Paul Bunnell test is negative, the original infection was probably more than a few weeks ago.

Glandular fever is also called infectious mononucleosis because of the large atypical mononuclear cells with an irregular nucleus which appear early on in the illness and may amount to up to 80% of the total white count of 10–20 × 10⁹/l, although more commonly 10–15%. In the very early stages of the illness, the white cell count may be normal or low. The Paul Bunnell test for antibodies is positive in about 60% of children during the first week of the illness but in others these antibodies only develop in the second or third week, so an early negative test should be repeated. This may remain positive for many weeks but may disappear by 2–4 weeks. A simple slide test, known as the 'monospot' test, is now commonly used as a screening procedure in infectious mononucleosis and is quicker and more sensitive than the Paul Bunnell reaction. Again this test may be negative early in the disease and if glandular fever is strongly suggested, it should be repeated.

Liver function tests are abnormal in >50% of cases, most often a mild increase in the transaminases, reflecting a derangement of hepatocellular function but less commonly there may be raised concentrations of alkaline phosphatase and bilirubin in the serum. There may be a clinical hepatitis in association with these biochemical findings, in which case the abnormality of liver function tests is more marked. Rarely, thrombocytopenia or a transient autoimmune haemolytic anaemia may occur and, historically, glandular fever was recognized as a cause of a false positive Wasserman reaction (a test for syphillis).

The importance of these investigations are that clinically this 'kissing disease' is very heterogenous, the commonest features being non-specific symptoms such as anorexia, malaise, fever and sore throat. However, clinical clues are that the spleen is often enlarged, there may be petechiae on the palate even in the absence of thrombocytopenia, and there is often a skin rash. If the illness is allowed to follow its natural course, a rash which may mimic measles, scarlet fever, purpura or urticaria, occurs in 10–15% of cases. However, if the child is given ampicillin to treat what was thought to be a bacterial tonsillitis, in over 90% of cases a skin rash appears within 2–3 days. This should not, however, be used as a diagnostic provocation test as laryngeal oedema may occur.

There are many rare complications of glandular fever which can mimic other diseases, including aseptic meningitis, Bell's palsy, a mild encephalitis or transverse myelitis, Guillain-Barré syndrome, myocarditis or arrhythmias, pneumonitis or orchitis. In some children, there is a prolonged period of convalescence with remission and relapse of malaise; if the initial diagnosis is not suggested by obvious features such as jaundice, splenomegaly or appropriate blood tests, chronic Epstein-Barr viral infection may be confused with chronic fatigue syndrome (ME).

Further reading

Campbell A G M, McIntosh N (eds) 1992 Forfar and Arneil's Textbook of paediatrics, 4th edn. Churchill Livingstone, Edinburgh, pp. 1422–1423
Editional 1985 Epstein-Barr virus and persistent malaise. Lancet i: 1017–1018
Editorial 1986 Ennervating illness and Epstein-Barr virus. Lancet ii: 141–142

Answer 11.6

1. Inborn error of metabolism
2. Ketonuria
   Reducing substances
   Organic aciduria
   Amino aciduria
   Urine pH

Discussion

The only obvious explanation for the seizures is hypoglycaemia (defined as a plasma glucose <2.2 mmol/l or a whole blood glucose <2.7 mmol/l). This is accompanied by a profound metabolic acidosis with compensatory respiratory alkalosis, explaining the hyperventilation. Sepsis is usually accompanied by hyperglycaemia (as part of the stress response) and fever. The combination of hypoglycaemia and severe metabolic acidosis strongly suggests a metabolic problem. Pituitary and adrenal insufficiency are possibilities but would usually be accompanied by electrolyte disturbances (hyponatraemia and hyperkalaemia with a pre-renal increase in urea). Hyperinsulinism is not usually associated with profound metabolic acidosis. The most likely explanation is an enzyme deficiency due to an inborn error of metabolism (e.g. glucose-6-phosphate deficiency in Type 1 glycogen storage disease, fructosaemia, galactosaemia, maple syrup urine disease, methyl malonic acidaemia, mitochondrial defects of fatty acid oxidation) but it is impossible to be more specific with the data available.

The presence of ketonuria excludes hyperinsulinism and defects of fatty acid oxidation. In other enzyme deficiencies, the acidosis is usually due to a combination of increased ketone bodies (as fatty acids are oxidized instead of glucose) and lactate (another alternative source of energy). Reducing substances in the urine, in the absence of glycosuria, would suggest galactosaemia (often precipitated by a trivial intercurrent infection in an infant who is not breast fed, as formula milks contain less lactose) or fructosaemia (50% of which present in the neonatal period). The dicarboxylic aciduria of fatty acid defects and methyl malonic aciduria would be detected by organic acid chromatography. Amino acid chromatography would show branched-chain amino acids in maple syrup urine disease. An appropriately acidic urine (pH 4−5) excludes renal bicarbonate loss as the cause of the acidosis, although this is not associated with hypoglycaemia.

Further reading

Campbell A G M, McIntosh N (eds) 1992 Forfar and Arneil's Textbook of paediatrics, 4th edn. Churchill Livingstone, Edinburgh, pp. 324−326
Milner A D, Hull D 1992 Hospital paediatrics, 2nd edn. Churchill Livingstone, Edinburgh, pp. 298−300, 437−438

Answer 11.7

1. Non-compliance with treatment

Discussion

Doses of 100−120 µg/m^2 of thyroxine replacement are usually required in early life (usually titrated to keep plasma thyroxine levels in the upper half of the normal range and the TSH levels within the normal range). The total T4 level at the upper limit of normal suggests that the dose of 25 μg is adequate to maintain a normal circulating thyroxine level. Why then is the TSH level high?

TSH controls the rate of release of thyroid hormones into the circulation; the principle thyroid hormone is thyroxine (T4) but the more potent tri-iodothyronine (T3) is also found in the plasma. The hormones circulate in the plasma bound to albumin and to an α-globulin known as thyroxine-binding globulin. In turn, circulating T4 exerts negative feedback on TSH release by the anterior pituitary.

The explanation of the data is that there is general background non-compliance with treatment so that there is no negative feedback inhibition of TSH release (normal range 0.1–4.3 mU/l) but the thyroxine is given in the few days immediately before the clinic attendance so that the T4 is within the normal range at the time of the blood test. The results cannot be explained by abnormalities of thyroid carrier proteins. These are rare in childhood but, for example, oestrogen therapy leads to an increase in thyroxine-binding globulin so that total T4 will appear to be high but free T4 and TSH levels will be normal and the patient may be clinically euthyroid. Decreased thyroxine-binding globulin may occur in nephrotic syndrome, cirrhosis and a very rare hereditary form of thyroid-binding globulin deficiency. These children have low total T4 levels, but again free T4 and TSH levels are normal and the child is clinically euthyroid.

Previously, thyroid function testing was confusing, involving a multiplicity of tests, many of which were indirect measures of thyroid function. Now, plasma TSH concentrations can be measured directly by radioimmunoassay and free T4 and T3 can be measured in addition to the total levels. Thyroxine replacement therapy should be monitored not only with plasma T4 and TSH levels but by growth velocity and bone age maturation. Clinical examination alone for signs of hypothyroidism or hyperthyroidism is insensitive for both initial diagnosis and assessing adequacy of thyroxine replacement.

The difficulty of diagnosing congenital hypothyroidism, the risk of permanent mental handicap following delayed presentation, and the incidence of 1 in 3500 live births have justified the incorporation of screening for congenital hypothyroidism within the original Guthrie test. This is done by using the blood spot to assay for high TSH levels. This will miss hypothyroidism due to hypothalamic or pituitary disease (in which TSH and T4 levels are both low) but this is a much rarer condition.

Answer 11.8

1. Liver failure
2. Reye's syndrome
   Aminoaciduria
   Fatty acid oxidation defect
   Sodium valproate therapy
   Gastrointestinal bleeding in presence of liver disease

Discussion

The child presents with a normal platelet count but a very high prolonged activated partial prothrombin time which assesses the intrinsic clotting pathway and is vitamin-K dependent. These clotting factors are synthesized largely in the liver. The extremely high ammonia level in the blood is consistent with failure of the urea cycle within the hepatocytes. You may not be expected to know the normal range of ammonia in the examination but, as a rough guide, a concentration >80 μmol/l is significantly abnormal outside the neonatal period. The most common explanation for the combination of hyperammonaemia and coagulopathy is liver failure in Reye's syndrome.

Three of the enzymes of the urea cycle are mitochondrial and while portions of the urea cycle exist in several tissues, it is only complete in the liver where urea is synthesized. In severe liver failure, hyperammonaemia may occur as a non-specific finding and may contribute to the encephalopathy of liver failure. However, it is a frequent finding in Reye's syndrome in the early stage of the illness, probably as a result of mitochondrial damage. The ammonia may fall towards normal levels 4-5 days into the illness. Great care must be taken in obtaining fresh samples for measuring blood ammonia levels and transporting these in a chilled container for rapid assay, as erroneously high values are common. However, these would not be associated with a coagulopathy.

Reye's syndrome is an acute encephalopathy which follows a prodromal illness and is accompanied by hepatocellular liver failure due to fatty infiltration. The onset of liver failure usually follows a mild respiratory illness or viral exanthema and vomiting is a common prodromal feature. Hepatomegaly is a frequent finding. Epidemiological associations have been made with therapeutic use of aspirin in children under 12 years, chickenpox or influenza, and inborn errors. Reye's syndrome has become much rarer since the product licence for the use of aspirin in children was amended.

Hyperammonaemia may result from a urea cycle disorder, the commonest of which is ornithine carbamoyl transferase deficiency (also known as ornithine transcarbamylase deficiency). In liver failure, plasma urea may actually fall as it can no longer be synthesized and plasma ammonia rises. Ammonia is then converted by an alternative pathway into orotic acid. In the presence of high ammonia, the finding of orotic acid in the urine therefore points to a urea cycle disorder. In a well child this may be suspected by a rise in plasma ammonia following a protein meal. Ornithine carbamoyl transferase deficiency is X-linked dominant and males are more severely affected than females.

In general, urea cycle deficiencies present with either an acute metabolic crisis, which may be precipitated by an increased protein intake or, in older infants, more gradual onset of poor feeding, vomiting, failure to thrive, lethargy and irritability. Liver failure and coagulopathy are not usually features of presentation and therefore urea cycle disorders are not an acceptable answer to question 2.

The organic acidurias — propionic, isovaleric and methylmalonic aciduria — may all present in this way. Urine should be collected for organic assay in any child who presents acutely with encephalopathy or liver failure and any child with a mental retardation of unknown cause. Many of the organic acidurias occur as a result of disorders of amino acid metabolism but there are other causes, e.g. diabetic ketoacidosis, glycogen storage disease Type 1, etc. Likewise, many of the amino acid disorders do not lead to organic aciduria. Most, but not all, organic acidurias are associated with metabolic acidosis. Similarly many, but not all, of the disorders of amino acid metabolism are associated with metabolic acidosis. Moreover, not all metabolic acidoses are associated with organic aciduria or amino aciduria. These overlaps between the different groups of conditions frequently lead to confusion. If there is diagnostic doubt in metabolic disorders, metabolic acidosis or mental retardation, blood and urine samples should both be obtained for examination of concentrations of amino acids and organic acids.

In fetal life there is a continuous supply of glucose across the placenta, but after birth fatty acids are a major fuel for cardiac and skeletal muscle both at rest and during aerobic exercise. This transition period is not normally stretched by the normal feeding regimens of newborn infants but as feeding times increase or during a catabolic illness or fasting, these enzymes can be overloaded as breakdown of fatty acids is increased and dicarboxylic acids accumulate. This is particularly likely to occur in an infant who has a deficiency or lack of one of the enzymes necessary for β-oxidation of fatty acids within the mitochondria. In general, the clinical manifestations are lethargy with nausea and vomiting, hypoglycaemia and a hepatic encephalopathy, and is very similar to Reye's syndrome. Abundant dicarboxylic aciduria is an important clue in distinguishing these disorders from classical Reye's syndrome.

Aminoaciduria such as hyperlysinaemia and hyperornithinaemia may present with acute liver failure.

There are a small number of autosomal recessive errors of pyrimidine metabolism which can present with raised ammonia, orotic aciduria and a megaloblastic anaemia.

Transient hyperammonaemia commonly follows the start of sodium valproate therapy, is usually a transient biochemical finding which is asymptomatic, and is not a reason to stop anticoagulant therapy. This is not related to severe liver failure. Liver failure is commoner if the child has several anticonvulsants or has an inborn error of metabolism and is more likely to occur within the first 3 months of therapy. There is not usually a gradual onset or warning but early signs which suggest withdrawal of anticonvulsants and checking of liver function tests are vomiting, lethargy and drowsiness.

Transient hyperammonaemia is sometimes seen in the neonatal period in infants receiving intravenous nutrition due to the high nitrogen load. Even in the preterm infant not receiving total parenteral nutrition, the liver enzymes may be sufficiently immature as to cause transient hyperammonaemia and this may be symptomatic. If treated vigorously the prognosis is excellent and there is no longterm liver or enzyme dysfunction.

A small amount of ammonia is formed in and absorbed from the gut but is not normally of any significance. However, excess ammonia is formed following gastrointestinal bleeding and if this occurs in the presence of a damaged liver, it is not taken up by the urea cycle and passes in the blood to the brain where it exacerbates hepatic encephalopathy. In order to avoid this complication, the gut is cleared of blood and protein contents with laxatives in the presence of liver failure.

The immediate management of all these conditions is similar and these are the steps of management of acute liver failure. If possible, the underlying cause should be treated, but this is often not immediately clear. If possible, drugs should be avoided as these may precipitate coma or a worsening of liver failure. Electrolyte imbalance should be corrected, intravenous vitamin K and fresh frozen plasma given to correct the coagulopathy, and intravenous glucose given to avoid hypoglycaemia. Initially the child should be kept nil by mouth apart from oral lactulose to clear the gut of any protein contents and/or blood. The use of oral neomycin to sterilize the gut is variable. Once an oral diet is resumed, this should be a low protein diet. Early discussion with a centre with experience in diagnosing rare metabolic problems is advised.

Further reading

Cowley H C, Webster N R 1993 Management of liver disease on the intensive care unit. Care of the Critically Ill 9: 122–127
Walter J H 1992 Metabolic acidosis in newborn infants. Archives of Disease of Childhood 67: 767–768

Answer 11.9

1. Salicyclate injestion

Metabolic acidosis
2. Forced alkaline diuresis

Discussion

There is a metabolic acidosis with a low normal $PaCO_2$, suggesting a compensatory respiratory alkalosis. The urine is appropriately acidic given the acidaemia of the blood. The very low urinary sodium (usually >30 mmol/l) and high urine osmolality suggest avid retention of sodium and water by the kidney. The blood sodium and osmolality are normal (normal range 275–290 mOsmol/kg). The most likely explanation for the urine results is shock causing pre-renal hypovolaemia. The most likely explanation for the combination of metabolic acidosis, shock, hyperglycaemia and prolonged prothrombin time is salicyclate ingestion. Most inborn errors of metabolism, which cause metabolic acidosis and shock, are associated with hypoglycaemia rather than hyperglycaemia. If heparin had been used in the syringe to obtain the arterial blood, this would prolong the partial prothrombin time but would have little effect on the prothrombin ratio.

Salicyclate poisoning has become less common in paediatrics since the withdrawal of a product licence for this analgesic in childhood (except for the treatment of chronic joint pain by an experienced rheumatologist). Aspirin in overdose acts as a respiratory stimulant, but alkalaemia is rarely seen in childhood as this only occurs in the early phase and is soon followed by metabolic acidosis. Respiratory acidosis is seen as a later feature when respiratory depression and coma supervene. Other clinical symptoms are nausea, vomiting, tinnitus and fever. There may be epigastric pain and vomiting. Despite the tendency for salicyclates in therapeutic dosage to cause gastric erosions, haematemesis very rarely occurs following overdosage and blood-stained gastric contents are seldom seen on gastric lavage. The prolonged prothrombin time is not a feature of diabetic ketoacidosis which would be the other major differential diagnosis of metabolic acidosis in conjunction with hyperglycaemia. In aspirin overdose, a purple–brown colour is seen on dipsticks used for the detection of phenylketonuria, and following boiling and acidification of urine, addition of ferric chloride gives a reddish-brown colour; a negative test with ferric chloride excludes aspirin poisoning.

The major differences between the two sets of results are that metabolic acidosis is largely corrected in the second set and urine is now alkaline with a higher urinary sodium and an osmolality which suggests that it is virtually isotonic with plasma. This girl has had a forced alkaline diuresis which is used in the treatment of moderate to severe aspirin overdose (salicyclate level at 4–6 h after ingestion of >650 mg/l, i.e. >4.7 mmol/l). This is achieved by infusing dextrose saline at 30 ml/kg/h and sodium bicarbonate at 1 mmol/kg, increasing gradually until the urine pH is 8. Alkalinizaton of the urine is more important than the induction of excessive urine flow. Higher salicyclate concentrations may require haemolysis or peritoneal dialysis.

Urine pH varies greatly with diet, but is usually acidic rather than alkaline (approx. 5–6). An acidic urine (<4.6) is always seen in metabolic acidosis unless the cause of the metabolic acidosis is renal tubular acidosis. Other causes of acidic urine are starvation leading to ketonuria, chronic respiratory acidosis and infected urine. An alkaline urine (>8) is a rarer finding but will occur with chronic respiratory alkalosis (unless there is profound hypokalaemia) and renal tubular acidosis and if the urine is infected with proteus or pseudomonas species. Metabolic alkalosis is less common than acidosis but may be seen with pyloric stenosis or as a result of iatrogenic alkalinization for salicyclate overdose or tumour lysis syndrome.

Further reading

Henry J, Volanz G 1984 ABC of poisoning. British Medical Association, London

Answer 11.10

1. Syndrome of inappropriate antidiuretic hormone secretion (SIADH)
2. Fluid restriction

Discussion

The data demonstrate this child has bacterial meningitis, SIADH leading to severe hyponatraemia and seizures. If the plasma and urine osmolalities had been normal, the most likely causes of the seizure would be a febrile convulsion (which is a common presentation of infants between 6 months and 2 years who have bacterial meningitis and up to 10% of these infants will have a further febrile convulsion while in hospital) or a seizure as a direct complication of the meningitic process.

Inappropiate secretion of antidiuretic hormone in children, i.e. not due to the normal stimuli of hyperosmolality or hypovolaemia, is seen in a variety of disorders:

a) increased hypothalamic production of antidiuretic hormone:

— intracranial disorders: infections (meningitis, encephalitis or abscess), vascular causes (subarachnoid haemorrhage or subdural haematoma), brain tumour;
— drugs: vincristine, cyclophosphamide, carbamazepine;
— pulmonary infections: pneumonia, tuberculosis.

b) exogenous administration of antidiuretic hormone:

— pitressin given to stop bleeding varices;
— theorectical risk of intranasal DDAVP (used to treat nocturnal enuresis).

Because of the effect of antidiuretic hormone on the collecting tubules (enhances renal water reabsorption), ingested water is retained resulting in dilutional hyponatraemia, hypo-osmolality and expansion of the body fluids. Oedema does not occur because it is always accompanied by an increase in total body water and sodium and in SIADH there is only an increase in total body water. If there is no water intake or water intake is restricted, water retention cannot occur and the excessive amounts of antidiuretic hormone can have no effect on the plasma sodium concentration or osmolality.

Two preconditions of the diagnosis of SIADH are that the child should not be overtly hypovolaemic and should not have received potent loop diuretics. The cardinal feature of SIADH is that the urine osmolality is inappropriately raised compared with the plasma osmolality. The urine osmolality need not itself be excessively high but the appropriate response to plasma hypo-osmolality is the excretion of a very dilute urine (with a lower osmolality than plasma in an effort to return the plasma osmolality to normal) and if the urine osmolality is greater than plasma in the presence of plasma hypo-osmolality, this is sufficient to diagnose SIADH.

It is important to understand that SIADH is an abnormality only of water excretion and renal function is otherwise unaffected. Clinical correlates of SIADH are fluid retention, weight gain, decreased urine output and an alteration of conscious level and possibly seizures due to the cerebral effects of hyponatraemia. However, there will be no rise in urea and creatinine as renal blood flow and glomerular filtration rate continue to be normal, and there is no hypertension because the increase in circulating volume activates volume receptors producing an increase in urinary sodium excretion (urinary sodium >20 mmol/l), despite the reduction in urine output. Similarly, oedema does not occur because sodium clearance is normal or increased and there is, therefore, no sodium retention and no increase in total body sodium, which usually accompanies oedema.

An essential step in SIADH is the retention of restricted water, leading to hypervolaemia. If the amount of water ingested is restricted, the adverse reaction of antidiuretic hormone on the plasma osmolality is avoided. This is most easily achieved by restricting total fluid intake to less than output (e.g. give two-thirds of the calculated maintenance) and this has the advantage that it corrects the electrolyte abnormalities slowly. If the plasma sodium is so low that seizures cannot be controlled, a more rapid correction can be achieved by producing a diuresis with frusemide and replacing the sodium lost in the resulting diuresis with 3% saline. For example, if after intravenous frusemide, there is a 1000 ml diuresis containing 150 mmol of sodium, these 150 mmol can be replaced in 300 ml 3% saline intravenously. The net effect is the loss of 700 ml of water with no change in sodium balance. SIADH must never be treated by giving sodium alone as this will be excreted in the urine (sodium clearance is already increased in SIADH) and as a result will produce no sustained rise in plasma sodium concentration.

The normal pulse, blood pressure and urea show that this child is not hypovolaemic and that fluid restriction is a safe treatment.

Paper 12 *QUESTIONS*

Question 12.1

A baby born at term to a healthy mother who had been on no medical treatment was found to have ambiguous genitalia. The infant was noted to have either a bifid scrotum or fused labia and gonads were palpable bilaterally within these perineal folds. The phallus was small and there was a perineal urethra. The following results were obtained:

Karyotype	46 XY
Plasma sodium	140 mmol/l
Plasma potassium	3.5 mmol/l
17 α-hydroxyprogesterone	Normal
Urinary steroid profile	Normal
Human chorionic gonadotrophin stimulation test:	
Pre-stimulation testosterone	1.8 mmol/l
Post-stimulation plamsa testosterone	1.8 nmol/l

Contrast radiology via the perineal urethra showed a vagina and uterus with a fistula between the vagina and urethra.

1. What is the most likely diagnosis?

Question 12.2

These are the ECG findings of a 7-year-old child during treatment for acute diabetic ketoacidosis (A) and a 10-year-old child on intensive care (B). C shows a normal trace from an 8-year-old child.

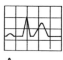
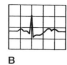
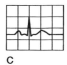

A   B   C

1. What do the ECG findings from the patient with diabetic ketoacidosis suggest?
2. What do the ECG findings from the patient with renal failure suggest?

Question 12.3

An 18-month-old boy, who had bacterial meningitis as a neonate, presents with a febrile convulsion. Lumbar puncture reveals turbid cerebrospinal fluid with the following results:

White cell count	42 000 polymorphs/μl
Protein	3.5 g/l
Glucose	0.5 mmol/l
Gram stain	Same Gram-negative organism as in the original episode of meningitis

1. What is the most likely pathogen in this case?
2. Give three problems associated with recurrent bacterial meningitis.

Question 12.4

An 18-month-old boy presented with a bruise on his thigh and a palpable haemoatoma over the quadriceps of his left leg. There was no family history of a bleeding disorder.

Haemoglobin	12.3 g/dl
Platelet count	300×10^9/l
Skeletal survey	Normal
Prothrombin time	12 s (control 12 s)
Partial thromboplastin time	130 s (control 45 s)
Thrombin time	15 s (control 15 s)

1. What is the most likely diagnosis?
2. What further test would you perform to confirm the diagnosis?

Question 12.5

Blood was taken from an infant in casualty. These results were obtained:

Plasma calcium	1.5 mmol/l
Plasma potassium	5.6 mmol/l
Haemoglobin	12 g/dl

The doctor had taken blood into a lithium heparin bottle and then poured some into an EDTA bottle to save time.

1. Has the doctor's short cut caused these abnormal results?

Question 12.6

These results were obtained from an 11-year-old boy with epigastric discomfort and severe diarrhoea:

Stool lipids | Increased
Fasting serum gastrin | 1750 pg/ml (normal 50–200 pg/ml)
Basal acid secretion | 65% of maximal acid output

1. What is the most likely diagnosis?
2. What is the cause of the diarrhoea?

Question 12.7

A baby is born at 31 weeks gestation following an antepartum haemorrhage. After 1 h he begins to grunt and develops an increasing oxygen requirement By 4 h the baby is intubated and ventilated on the following settings:

Rate | 40/min
I:E ratio | 1:1
Pressure | 24/4 cmH$_2$O
FiO$_2$ | 0.75

The infant looks pink and settled and is not hypotensive. The most recent blood gas results from the umbilical catheter are:

pH | 7.19
PaO$_2$ | 5.8 kPa
PaCO$_2$ | 8.5 kPa

1. What is the most likely cause for the infant requiring ventilation?
2. What two actions would you take?

Question 12.8

A breast-fed term infant is noted to be jaundiced at 1 day old. Both parents are caucasian; the father is blood group A Rhesus positive and the mother O, Rhesus negative. There is no family history of jaundice and the mother's anti-D antibody titres remained unchanged during pregnancy.

Urinalysis | Negative for bilirubin
Total plasma bilirubin | 112 μmol/l

Conjugated bilirubin   11 μmol/l
Direct Coombs' test   Negative

1. What are the two most likely diagnoses?
2. What two further haematological investigations would you request?

Question 12.9

This is a family genogram.

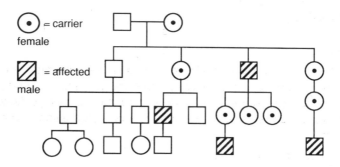

1. Suggest two possible disorders that would be consistent with this family.

Question 12.10

A baby girl is born at 34 weeks gestation with a birth weight of 1.4 kg (below 3rd centile) and a head circumference of 31 cm (50th centile). The father is 5'10" and the mother 5'5". At 3-month follow-up, the girl weighs 4 kg (still below 3rd centile). She is taking 3 fl oz of formula milk, four times a day. At 10 months of age the child's weight remains below the 3rd centile. On examination there are no abnormalities. Investigation shows the following results:

Plasma alkaline phosphatase	1800 IU/l
Plasma alanine aminotransferase	15 IU/l
Plasma bilirubin	8 μmol/l
Total plasma calcium	2.25 mmol/l
Plasma phosphate	1.8 mmol/l
X-ray of left wrist	Normal for age

3 months later, the child's alkaline phosphatase is 400 IU/l without any treatment.

1. What is the most likely cause of her poor weight gain?
2. What is your biochemical diagnosis?

Paper 12 ANSWERS

Answer 12.1

1. Testicular dysgenesis
Combined Leydig and Sertoli cell failure

Combined deficiency of testosterone and Müllerian inhibitory factor

Male pseudohermaphrodite
Incompletely virilized male

Discussion

This infant with ambiguous genitalia is an incompletely virilized male. This is indicated by the normal male karyotype and the fact that both gonads are palpable in the labio-scrotal folds; these are almost always testes. The cause of an incompletely virilized genetic male (sometimes called male pseudohermaphrodite) are:

— an enzyme defect in testosterone;
— testicular dysgenesis;
— androgen insensitivity of target organs.

The failure of any rise in plasma testosterone following HCG (normally there should be a rise of 2 nmol/l or more) suggests that the problem is one of testosterone production and not androgen insensitivity due to target organ failure. If the diagnosis were simply a defect in testosterone biosynthesis, there would be inadequate virilization but no persistence of female organs internally. The only explanation for the data above is testicular dysgenesis with a combination of Leydig cell failure (failure to produce testosterone and a lack of virilization), and Sertoli cell failure (failure in production of Müllerian inhibitory factor, with consequent preservation of uterus and vagina).

In cases of neonatal ambiguous genitalia, no attempt should be made to guess the sex in the immediate neonatal period. The parents should be told that a definitive diagnosis will be arrived at as soon as possible, almost always within a week or 2, and they should defer choosing a name until the sex of rearing has been decided. An infant's sex can be defined as genetic sex (XX for a female, XY for a male), gonadal sex (the presence of ovaries or testes, or both in a true haemaphrodite), phenotypic sex (the internal and external genitalia) and finally functional sex (determined by a combination of the above but particularly by phallic size as the success of reconstructive vaginal surgery is much greater than that of the penis). The final decision may have to be deferred until a trial of testosterone therapy is used to establish whether the phallus has the capacity for androgen responsiveness and acceptable future growth. The only other investigation which is likely to take some time is of androgen-binding studies performed on genital skin fibroblasts and used to test for end-organ insensitivity. Androgen insensitivity may not present as ambiguous genitalia but may become apparent in young adult life when a girl fails to menstruate. If the chromosomes show a normal male karyotype, the diagnosis is one of complete androgen insensitivity (testicular feminization syndrome).

Further reading

Campbell A G M, McIntosh N (eds) 1992 Forfar and Arneil's Textbook of paediatrics, 4th edn. Churchill Livingstone, Edinburgh, pp. 1071–1072, 1103, 1137

Answer 12.2

1. Hypokalaemia
2. Hyperkalaemia

Discussion

Hypokalaemia produces fairly non-specific ECG changes. However, when the serum potassium is <2.5 mmol/l, the following ECG changes may be found:

— prominent U-wave. There is apparent prolongation of the Q–T interval but, in fact, a long Q–U interval is present;
— flat or diphasic T-waves;
— ST segment depression.

With further lowering of the serum potassium, the P–R interval may be prolonged and sino-atrial block may occur.

All these ECG features of hypokalaemia may be found in left ventricular hypertorphy with strain. Both hypokalaemia and digitalis produce ST segment depression. However, digitalis produces a short Q–T interval and usually no prominence of the U-wave.

ECG features typical of hyperkalaemia are best seen in the left precordial leads. These include:

— tall 'tented' T-waves;
— prolongation of the QRS duration (intraventricular block);
— prolongation of the P–R interval;
— disappearance of the P-wave;
— wide, bizarre, diphasic QRS complex (Sine wave).

Answer 12.3

1. Escherichia coli

2. Dural sinus
   Otitis media
   Mastoiditis
   Sinusitis
   Skull fracture
   Intraventricular shunt

Discussion

The most likely pathogen is *E. coli*, which is rarely seen as a cause of meningitis outside the neonatal period. This child has recurrent meningitis and he either is extraordinarily unlucky or, more likely, has an underlying anatomical or microbiological reason for recurrent meningitis:

a) association with the presence of a congenital dural sinus, which leads to communication between the subarachnoid space and the overlying skin either at the level of the lumbar spine or more rarely at the occipital spine. A lumbar dural sinus is particularly likely to become contaminated by faecal material from the baby's nappy and *E.coli* is a likely organism. If the sinus were higher, e.g. a cervical dural sinus, skin contaminants (Gram-positive cocci such as *Staphylococcus aureus, Staphylococcus epidermidis* or Gram-positive bacilli such as diptheroides) would be possible causes;

b) if the child were older and had recurrent purulent sinusitis, *Streptococcus milariae* may cause recurrent meningitis or a cerebral abscess in association with frontal sinusitis;

c) if the child had had a neurosurgical procedure or had been born with spina bifida, then staphylococcal species (either *Staphylococcus aureus* or *epidermidis*) would be likely causes of recurrent ventriculitis or meningitis;

d) certain forms of immunodeficiency (children with severe combined immunodeficiency homozygous for a deficiency in adenosine deaminase) are particularly vulnerable to type A meningococcal disease, which is otherwise rare in the UK, although seen in epidemics in the Middle East. Splenectomy is associated with increased risk of infection with *Streptococcus pneumoniae, Haemophilus influenzae* and *Neisseria meingitidis*, all three of which are causes of bacterial meningitis.

If this had been the child's first episode of meningitis, at 18 months of age the commonest cause of bacterial meningitis is *Haemophilus influenzae*. In this case, if there is another family member under the age of 3 years, then all 'kissing contacts' under the age of 5 years should be given rifampicin prophylaxis. In the case of meningococcal disease, 2 days of rifampicin 10 mg/kg b.d. should be given to all 'kissing contacts' as soon as possible, irrespective of their age.

The commonest associations with recurrent bacterial meningitis are:

— a dural sinus, either lumbosacral or occipital;
— chronic or recurrent otitis media, mastoiditis or sinusitis;
— an undiagnosed skull fracture with a dural tear leading to chronic CSF leakage (CSF otorrhoea or rhinorrhoea);

— presence of ventriculo-cardiac or ventriculo-peritoneal shunts to relieve hydrocephalus carry a risk of recurrent ventriculitis and meningitis, as these are foreign bodies which may be colonized in particular with *Staphylococcus epidermidis*.

Answer 12.4

1. Haemophilia
2. Specific assays of factors VIII, IX and XI

Discussion

With an isolated prolongation of partial prothrombin time in a well child with a haematoma, haemophilia is the most likely diagnosis. Family history may reveal a sex-linked pattern of inheritance. However, the family history may be negative owing to a predominance of females in successive generations, or the high rate of spontaneous mutations.

This child has moderate (2%) factor VIII activity (haemophilia A). The age and type of presentation correlates well with the level of factor VIIIc in a particular patient. Patients with levels <1% are severely affected and can present in early infancy with easy bruising or spontaneous haemarthroses when they become more mobile. The bruising may be confused with non-accidental injury. Severe manifestations, including intracranial haemorrhage, can occur following traumatic delivery. Recurrent painful haemarthroses and muscle haematomas often dominate the clinical course.

Haematuria is quite common, but gastrointestinal haemorrhage less so. Operative and post-traumatic haemorrhage may be life threatening. Interestingly, patients do not usually bleed excessively from cuts or from mucosal surfaces unless raw areas exist (e.g. tooth sockets following extraction).

Further reading

Campbell A G M, McIntosh N (eds) 1992 Forfar and Arneil's Textbook of paediatrics, 4th edn. Churchill Livingstone, Edinburgh, pp. 950–952

Answer 12.5

1. No

Discussion

This child was suffering from hypocalcaemia. The lithium heparin bottle is the correct bottle for routine biochemistry. Serious errors can arise if blood is poured from one container to another. Results may show hyperkalaemia and hypocalcaemia if blood had been taken into an 'EDTA' bottle for haematological investigations, and some then poured into a lithium heparin bottle for routine biochemistry.

The anticoagulant action of oxalate and of sequestrene (EDTA — ethylenediamene tetraacetate) depends on precipitation or chelation, respectively, of calcium. This invalidates results of calcium estimation and may cause a low calcium level to be recorded. EDTA is usually in the form of its potassium salt which may cause 'apparent' hyperkalaemia. Such mistakes could have serious consequences.

Further reading

Zilva J F, Pannell P R, Mayne P D 1989 Clinical chemistry in diagnosis and treatment.

Answer 12.6

1. Zollinger–Ellison syndrome
2. Low intestinal pH produced by sustained acid hypersecretion

Discussion

Zollinger–Ellison syndrome encompasses severe peptic ulceration, hypersecretion of gastric acid, and an islet cell tumour of the pancreas. Prolonged high plasma gastrin concentrations cause an increase of the parietal cell mass with consequent high basal and maximal acid secretion.

The majority of patients have aggressive peptic ulceration. The second major symptom is diarrhoea and this may occassionally be the only presenting syndrome. Peptic ulcers may occur in the duodenum, the stomach or oesophagus.

The diarrhoea is unlikely to be due to hypergastrinaemia itself, for diarrhoea does not occur in patients with high gastrin levels from other causes, such as those with pernicious anaemia. The low pH produced by sustained acid hypersecretion denatures pancreatic enzymes, causing steatorrhoea and precipitates bile salts, causing bile salt malabsorption, which in turn promotes water secretion by the colon.

Further reading

Milla P J, Muller D P R 1988 Harries' paediatric gastroenterology, 2nd edn. Churchill Livingstone, Edinburgh, pp. 519–520

Answer 12.7

1. Respiratory distress syndrome
   Idiopathic respiratory distress syndrome

Surfactant deficiency
Hyaline membrane disease
2. Increase the inspired oxygen
Increase the ventilator rate

Increase the inspiratory pressure

Discussion

There are many possible causes for respiratory distress but the most likely in a preterm infant is surfactant deficiency leading to hyaline membrane disease. This disorder affects 80% of infants born at 28 weeks gestation and 50% of infants at 32 weeks and is more likely if the infant becomes cold or acidotic (e.g. as a result of hypotension following a large antepartum haemorrhage). Although the infant may manage initially, the lack of surfactant leads to respiratory distress (tachypnoea, expiratory grunting, intercostal recession and cyanosis in air). Onset >8 h after birth suggests an alternative diagnosis.

Surfactant, a natural mixture of phospholipid and protein released from the type 2 pneumocytes, is a surface tension lowering agent which increases lung compliance and prevents smaller alveoli coalescing into larger neighbouring alveoli. Surfactant deficiency is associated with stiff lungs, increased work of breathing, and hypoxia due to ventilation-perfusion mismatch, decreased alveolar surface area and increased thickness of the alveolar-capillary membrane.

There are a number of possible explanations for these blood gases in an infant who appears pink. The sample may be venous if the umbilical catheter is in the vein rather than the artery. If the catheter is in the umbilical artery, it should be sited below the renal vessels or just above the diaphragm. In either case, the tip will lie below the point where the ductus arteriosus enters the aorta. A sample of postductal blood may be more hypoxic than that supplying the face and lips if there is an element of persistent fetal circulation complicating the hyaline membrane disease and leading to extracardiac right-to-left shunting. Finally, if the baby has suffered significant blood loss, cyanosis is more difficult to detect clinically in the face of anaemia as there is less circulating deoxyhaemoglobin for any given oxygen saturation. However, none of these possibilities explains the hypercapnia. There may have been a transcription error — perhaps the PaO_2 is 8.5 and the $PaCO_2$ 6.1?

Assuming the blood gas result is genuine, the infant is hypoxic (the clinical observation that 'he looks pink' is not sufficiently reliable in intensive care) and has a significant respiratory acidosis, both of which will tend to cause pulmonary vasoconstriction and a worsening of the respiratory distress. After checking that the baby's chest is moving, breath sounds are equal and there is no pneumothorax on transillumination, the correct action is to increase the FiO_2 to 0.85, to improve oxygenation, and increase the ventilator rate to 60/min to increase the minute volume and blow off more CO_2. This combination is preferable to simply increasing the inspiratory pressures as this will increase the risk of barotrauma and air leak. To give alkali would be inappropriate as the acidosis is predominantly a respiratory acidosis. A blood gas should be repeated after 20 min.

Answer 12.8

1. ABO incompatibility or spherocytosis
2. Maternal haemolysins
   Neonatal blood film

Discussion

The early age of onset of a significant level of jaundice in an infant who is not preterm is against physiological or breast-milk jaundice. The cause must be a haemolytic process as the bilirubin is almost all unconjugated; the 'acholuric' urine confirms this. The infant may be Rhesus positive (the father may be either heterozygous or homozygous for the Rhesus antigen) but the lack of a rising titre of Rhesus antibody in the mother suggests she has not been sensitized. If Rhesus incompatiblity were the cause, the Coombs' test would be strongly positive.

The infant may be group O or A (the alleles for the AB system of antigens are co-dominant and the father may be heterozygous or homozygous for group A, so it is impossible to be certain about the infant's ABO group) but if group A, an ABO incompatibility is possible. The mother's blood will contain anti-A antibody but this is usually an IgM which cannot cross the placenta (otherwise fetal haemolysis due to ABO incompatibility would be relatively common). However, some women produce an anti-A IgG antibody, which can cross the placenta, and if the infant's red cells carry the A antigen, haemolysis results. The direct Coombs' test is often only weakly positive or negative. Unlike Rhesus disease, ABO incompatibility does not seem to worsen with each pregnancy but, on the other hand, the first pregnancy can be affected.

Half of all cases of spherocytosis present in the neonatal period as haemolytic jaundice and half of these have no family history (the inheritance is autosomal dominant with variable severity). The cause of the jaundice is splenic consumption of red cells due to an erythrocyte membranopathy and therefore the Coombs' test, which implies an immune aetiology, is negative.

Maternal haemolysins (significant titres of anti-A IgG) should be sought and a blood film requested, recognizing that spherocytes are a relatively common finding on the blood film of a healthy neonate. The definitive test for spherocytes is the osmotic fragility test (the spherocytes are more likely to lyse in a saline solution than normal biconcave erythrocytes) but this is not completely reliable until after 3 months of age.

Answer 12.9

1. Retinitis pigmentosa

Ocular albinism
Nephrogenic diabetes insipidus
Haemophilia
Glucose-6-phosphate dehydrogenase deficiency
Colour blindness

Oculocerebrorenal syndrome
Duchenne muscular dystrophy
Hunter's syndrome

Discussion

The pedigree is that of an X-linked recessive trait in which affected males *do* survive to reproduce. As there are no structural genes other than those determining sexual development on the Y chromosome, sex-linkage is effectively the same as X-linked inheritance. An X-linked recessive trait is one which is due to an abnormal gene on the X chromosome and therefore the females are carriers and the males are affected. The affected males are hemizygous and because they possess only one X chromosome are invariably affected by the disorder, whilst the carrier females are heterozygous, with two X chromosomes and are usually perfectly healthy. X-linked disorders are also transmitted by affected males to their daughters unless the disorder is so severe that affected males do not survive to have children. Haemophilia is an example of an X-linked recessive disorder in which, because of improvements in medical treatment and transfusion products, affected males may now survive into adult life. If an affected male survives to reproductive age and marries a normal female, all his daughters will be carriers and all his sons will be normal. If a woman who is a carrier marries a normal male, then half her sons will be affected and half her daughters will be carriers like herself.

In some X-linked conditions, there may be only one affected boy in a family which does not allow depiction of the pedigree. Such a sporadic case may be the result of a new mutation on the affected boy's X chromosome and in such cases recurrrence would not occur in other family members. It is also possible that the mother is a carrier and by chance alone the mutant gene has not been transmitted to any of her male offspring. In one-third of isolated cases of Duchenne muscular dystrophy, the mutation occurs in the affected boy and in the other two-thirds of cases the mother is the carrier. It is of vital importance to determine if the mother is a carrier and with gene probes in some disorders it is possible to demonstrate unequivocally whether or not the parent is a carrier.

The most likely X-linked recessive disorders to give rise to the pedigree shown are those in which children survive into adult life. As mentioned above, haemophiliacs may now survive to reproductive age whereas in Duchenne muscular dystrophy, the disorder is so severe that affected males do not survive to have children and therefore would be unlikely to give rise to this pedigree.

Further reading
  Campbell A G M, McIntosh N (eds) 1992 Forfar & Arneil's Textbook of
  paediatrics, 4th edn. Churchill Livingstone, Edinburgh, pp. 71–74

Answer 12.10

1. Inadequate calorie intake
2. Transient hyperphosphatasaemia of infancy

Discussion

This girl was born asymmetrically growth retarded, with a normal-sized head
but light for gestational age. This is the commonest type of growth retardation
and is usually due to placental disease with onset in the third trimester.
Intrauterine infections, chromosomal disorder and several non-chromosomal
syndromes (e.g. Russell–Silver syndrome) cause symmetrical growth
retardation and onset is much earlier in pregnancy. In asymmetrical growth
retardation, there is commonly catch-up growth in the first 6 months of life with
'physiological up-regulation' as the infant's weight crosses the centiles, an
adequate source of nutrition after birth releasing growth from the in utero
placental constraint. This is particularly likely in this case as the parents' heights
are both well within the normal range. A mid-parental centile can be calculated
for any child by taking both parents' heights and, in the case of a girl, adjusting
them and plotting them as for an 18-year-old on a female centile curve. This is
achieved by subtracting 5" or 12 cm from the father's height and in this case this
gives heights for both parents of 5'5", which is almost the 50th centile for an
adult woman. The confidence limits for this prediction are ± 8 cm (2.5").

The normal range for milk intake varies with age, rising after birth to a
maximum of 150–225 ml/kg body weight/day at 1 month, and falling gradually
to 100–175 at 6 months. This infant has an intake at 3 months of age of 12 fl
oz/day (1 fl oz = 28 ml) and this is therefore well below normal for an infant of 4
kg. The commonest cause of failure to thrive at all ages is inadequate intake.
This may be because insufficient food is offered (either through ignorance or
deliberate neglect) or because of poor feeding practices in an inexperienced
young parent, a fussy eater or anorexia due to a systemic disease. Other
causes are legion but can be most logically thought of in order as food passes
down the gut into the intestinal tract: chronic vomiting or severe reflux, small
bowel malabsorption, increased energy requirements (increased metabolic
rate in thyrotoxicosis or increased work of breathing in a preterm infant with
respiratory failure), inadequate utilization for growth of appropriately absorbed
calories (endocrine diseases leading to short stature).

The child has a raised alkaline phosphatase (normal ranges vary with age
and laboratory but the maximum is never >1100 IU/l at any age, including early
infancy and puberty), with normal calcium, phosphate, liver function tests and
radiology. Transient hyperphosphatasaemia of infancy is suggested by the
very high alkaline phosphatase activity with otherwise normal investigations,

which returns to within the normal range usually within 3 months without any therapy. There is an atypical isoenzyme pattern and although the child is usually not perfectly healthy, this enzyme level is totally unrelated to the condition for which the child is being investigated.

Free (ionized) calcium is less than total calcium because calcium binds to albumin. If an albumin result is given in addition to the total calcium, a corrected calcium can be calculated by subtracting the albumin concentration from 40, multiplying by 0.02 and adding this to the quoted calcium. The calcium is only low in this example because of the low albumin. The free ionized calcium would be normal.

The changes in calcium, phosphate and alkaline phosphatase in disorders of bone metabolism in childhood are:

	Plasma Calcium	Plasma Phosphate	Plasma Alkaline Phosphatase
Rickets	Low/normal	Low	↑
Primary hyperparathyroidism	↑	Low	↑
Secondary hyperparathyroidism	↓	↓ (if the cause is rickets) ↑ (if the cause is chronic renal failure)	↑
True hypoparathyroidism	↓	↑	Normal
Pseudo-hypoparathyroidism	Low	↑	Normal
Pseudo-pseudohypoparathyroidism	Normal	Normal	Normal
Fanconi's syndrome	Normal	Low	Normal
Vitamin D resistant rickets	Low	Low	↑
Idiopathic hypercalcaemia of infancy	↑	Normal	Normal
Sarcoidosis	↑	Low	↑

Of these, rickets is the commonest, and may be due to a diet deficient in vitamin D or malabsorption of vitamin D in small bowel disease and biliary disease (vitamin D is fat soluble). Rickets may manifest during puberty when there is increased requirements. Hypophosphataemic rickets is almost always due to increased urinary loss but in a preterm infant, especially on unsupplemented formula, dietary intake of phosphate may be inadequate and biochemical and even radiological rickets may result.

INDEX